Modern Ketogenic Diet

Using the High-Fat And Low-Carb Hack Through The Keto Diet To Shred Fat And Feel Healthy Again (Rapid Weight Loss, Meal Plans, Healthier Lifestyle)

Elliot Cutting

Table of Contents

Introduction: The Keto Diet

Most people shorten the Ketogenic diet down and call it the "Keto diet." This word was created because while following this diet, your body creates fuel molecules called *Ketones*. Ketones get used as an alternate source of fuel for our bodies and the body uses these when its glucose supply gets low.

If you don't eat many carbs, your body will produce *Ketones*. This holds true if your protein intake is kept at moderate levels. If you eat too much protein, the body could turn it into sugar.

Your liver can create Ketones from the fat that has been stored in your body. The body will then use the Ketones for fuel for several parts of the body including the brain. The sad part is that our brains can't run off fuel we get from fat. It only gets fuel from glucose or *Ketones*.

While doing a Ketogenic diet, your whole body will change its fuel supply and be able to run entirely off of fat. This causes your insulin level to drop and your body to burn more fat. Your body will be accessing the fat that it has stored over the years and begin to burn it. This is a great diet if you are trying to lose weight and on top of that there are other benefits such as better mental awareness, steady energy supply, and less hunger.

Low Carbs

The only way that this diet will work correctly is by eating a very small amount of carbs. The fewer carbs you eat, the better your chances of losing weight. A Keto diet is very strict with low-carbs. You will only be able to eat 20 grams or less of net carbs every day.

Once you have achieved your weight loss goals, you can start to increase the number of carbs you eat. This will need to be done slowly so that you don't end up gaining the weight you lost.

Covering The Basics

It is a must that you follow this diet firmly in order to get better and faster results.

In theory, a Ketogenic diet is simple—low-carbs, high fat. This doesn't exactly tell you what you can and can't eat. There is a complete list of foods you can eat later on in the book, but for now here is a quick overview:

- Meats including organ meat.
- Fish and seafood
- Heavy fats such as bacon fat, tallow, butter, olive oil, coconut oil, ghee, and lard.
- Eggs
- Berries like blueberries, strawberries, and raspberries.
- Nonstarchy vegetables—all the leafy greens you care to eat.

Your typical day could look something like this:

- Breakfast could include bacon and eggs.
- Lunch could include a cup of bone broth with a chicken salad.
- Dinner might consist of a steak, side of veggies, and a dessert that is Keto-friendly.

Some people have to snack between meals. If you are like this, good choices are meat sticks, broth, cheese sticks, celery sticks, and nuts. You have to watch how many snacks you eat since these will make your total calorie count go up.

The Keto diet is very easy to personalize and you have the ability to experiment and figure out what will work best for you due to the various food options. Some people may realize that they need more fats in their diet, and others might be able to eat fewer carbs.

Ketosis

Let's take a closer look at it and figure out what it actually is. Ketosis is a natural state that the body goes into when it is fueled by fat. This will happen when you fast or follow a strict low-carb diet such as the Keto diet.

There are several benefits in allowing your body to get into Ketosis, these being increased health, performance, and weight loss. There are some side effects to consider just like anything else such as if you have type 1 diabetes or other diseases, too much Ketosis could be dangerous.

Once your body gets into Ketosis, it produces *Ketones*. As stated above, these small molecules can be used as fuel for the body. The liver converts fat into *Ketones* and releases them into the bloodstream. The body will then use them like glucose.

How to Get into Ketosis

Our bodies can get into Ketosis in two different ways; fasting or a Ketogenic diet. With either one of these ways, the body has limited sources of glucose, causing the body to switch and use fat for fuel. When the hormone insulin gets low, the body will increase its fat burning properties. This means your body now has access to all of your stored fat and melts it.

Scientifically proven, fasting will create ketosis in the body fast than the Keto diet, however most people decide to do the Keto diet because it can be eaten for an indefinite amount of time and you don't have to worry about hunger pains and food time management.

Fuel for Our Brains

Most people think the brain needs carbs for fuel. The brain actually can't burn carbs when you eat them, but if carbs aren't available, it burns Ketones.

This is needed for basic human survival. Because our bodies can only store carbs for one or two days, the brain will just shut down after several days without food. Alternatively, it would begin converting muscle protein into glucose fast in order to keep working. This is not very effective. This means we will waste away quickly. If this is the way the body actually works, then the human race would not have survived before food became available all day and every day.

The human body has evolved in order to work smarter. Normally, the body will have stored enough fat so that someone could survive a few weeks without eating anything at all. Ketosis a process of survival that happens to make sure our brains can run on fat stores.

Ketosis and Ketoacidosis

There are a lot of misconceptions about Ketosis. The main one is thinking it is the same thing as Ketoacidosis. Ketoacidosis is a rare but dangerous condition that happens to people who have type 1 diabetes. Sometimes even health care professionals mix these two things up. It might be because the names are very similar, and there isn't a lot of knowledge between the differences.

Ketosis is a natural state for the body, and our bodies control it all by itself. Ketoacidosis is a malfunction in the body where it creates an excessive and unregulated amount of Ketones. This could cause symptoms like stomach pain, nausea, and vomiting, which can be followed by confusion and even a coma. This requires urgent medical treatment and could end up being fatal.

So before someone gets this diet confused when you're having a conversation about it, you won't freak out and you will know exactly what they're talking about.

Reaching Optimal Level of Ketosis

This is the point that everybody who does the Ketogenic diet wants to get to. When you have reached the optimal level of Ketosis, your body will begin to burn fat at the best speed. To reach this level of Ketosis, you have to follow a low-carb, high-fat diet, as we stated above. You need to keep your macros at their optimal range. There aren't any specific tricks that will help you do this, just following the steps in this book and experiencing the diet for yourself will leave you with the answers you need.

Here are the different Ketone levels that you might have:

- Less than 0.5 means you haven't reached Ketosis yet.
- A level between 0.5 and 1.5 is a light level of Nutritional Ketosis. You might lose some weight, but you aren't at the optimal level.
- Levels around 1.5 to 3 is considered to be at the optimal level and is best for losing the most weight.
- Levels that are over 3 aren't needed. High levels don't help you at all. It might harm you because it means you aren't eating enough food.

Most people think they have been eating a strict Keto diet but when they measure their blood Ketone levels, they get surprised. Once they measure their levels and they are around 0.2 or 0.5, they realize they aren't near their sweet spot, and they get discouraged.

The trick of getting past this plateau is you have to stick to low-carb sources but also make sure you aren't eating too much protein. Your protein intake doesn't need to be higher than your fat intake. Yes, we have stated that protein doesn't affect your glucose levels as carbs will, but if you consume too many, especially if you eat more protein than fats, this will affect your glucose, effecting your optimal Ketosis.

The trick to working around this is eating more fat. You could easily do this by adding a big dollop of herbed butter to the top of your steak. This may help you not eat as much because fats fill you up quite easily.

Drinking a cup of bulletproof coffee can keep you from getting hungry and eating too much protein. This is simple to do; you just need to add a tablespoon of butter or coconut oil to your coffee every morning.

How to Measure Ketosis

There are many ways you can figure out if you have reached Ketosis. The first way is by measuring Ketones in your blood. This means you will have to buy a meter and prick your finger just like you would to measure blood sugar.

There are many reasonably priced gadgets out there, and it only takes a few seconds to find out what your blood Ketone level is. Most people don't want to go to this extreme just to find out what their Ketone level is, but is the most accurate and effective.

You will need to measure your blood Ketones first thing every morning on a fasted stomach. You can look at the levels we listed earlier to figure out if you are in Ketosis.

These meters measure the amount of BHB that's in your blood. This is the main Ketone that is present in the blood when you are in Ketosis. The biggest problem with this method is having to draw blood.

These kits will cost around $30 to $40 and might cost around $5 for every test. This is the reason most people that decide to test this way, just perform a test each week or so.

We've covered the most expensive way to figure out if you are in Ketosis but there are seven other ways to tell if you are in Ketosis.

1. Bad breath

    This doesn't sound pleasant but people have often stated that they have bad breath when they have reached Ketosis. This is a normal side effect. People have stated that their breath will smell fruitier.

    This is caused by elevated Ketone levels. The big culprit is the Ketone acetone that the body excretes through your breath and urine. You might not like the idea of having bad breath; but it is a great way to know if you are in

Ketosis. Most people will brush their teeth more often or chew some sugar-free gum.

2. Weight loss

   This is the best way to tell if you are in Ketosis. When you first start the Keto diet, you will see a quick drop in weight, but this is normally just water weight. When you experience another drop in weight, this will be your fat stores being burnt. This is another way to know you are in Ketosis.

3. Ketones in your breath and urine

   If you don't like having to prick your finger, you can measure blood Ketones by using a breath analyzer. This monitors acetone, which is one of the three Ketones that will be in your book when you reach Ketosis.

   This will let you know when your Ketone levels have hit Ketosis since acetone only leaves the body when you have reached nutritional Ketosis. These breath analyzers are fairly accurate but not as accurate as the blood monitor.

   Another way you could check for Ketosis is checking for Ketones in your urine every day using special indicator strips. This is a cheap and fast method you can use to assess what your Ketones levels are every day. These methods are not very reliable.

4. Appetite suppression

   Most people report their hunger will decrease when following a Keto diet. The reasons behind this are still being studied. It is thought that the reduction in hunger is due to the increase in protein and vegetable consumption, as well as a change in hunger hormones. The Ketones might also affect how your brain reacts to hunger.

5. Better focus and energy

Some people have reported feeling sick, tired, or having brain fog when they first start the Keto diet. This is called the Keto flu. People that follow this diet for a long time have reported having better energy and increased focus. Your body will need time to adapt to this new diet. Once you hit Ketosis, your brain begins to burn Ketones for energy. This could take a week or two for it to start happening.

6. Short-term fatigue

Once your body starts making the switch to Keto, it might cause weakness and fatigue. This makes it hard for some people to stick with this diet. This side effect is normal, but it is a way to know that you are hitting Ketosis.

This crappy feeling might last for one week or one month before you actually hit full Ketosis. You can reduce this feeling by taking electrolyte supplements.

7. Short-term performance decrease

Just like this point before, the fatigue may cause a decrease in exercise performance. This is caused by the glycogen stores in your muscles being reduced; this gives you the fuel you need to get through high-intensity exercises. After a week or two, your performance levels will return to normal.

Keto Diet Versus the Atkins Diet

These are the two most popular diets that will reduce your intake of carbs drastically, but let's look at how they compare to each other in terms of results, safety, and difficulty.

The Atkins diet and the Ketogenic diet would be tied in a race for the most popular low-carb diets. Both don't just cut back on carbs, like donuts, cupcakes, and cookies, but they also get rid of some veggies, and most fruits. They limit the number of carbs so much that it makes you enter into Ketosis; this makes the body burn fat for fuel once your glucose stores have been depleted. Ketosis plays a huge role in both these diets, and it can also affect how easy it is to stick with them.

Let's go through the Atkins diet quickly. It was introduced in 1972 by Robert Atkins, who was a cardiologist. The original diet, that is now called Atkins 20, had four phases. The first phase had a lot of restrictive rules.

Proteins and fats in the Atkins diet are both fair game but carbs are extremely restricted to around 20 and 25 grams of net carbs. This is the total carbs minus the dietary fiber. All of these carbs need to come from veggies, cheese, seeds, and nuts. This phase will last until you are about 15 pounds away from your goal weight.

Phase two brings your carb amount to about 25 to 50 grams, and you can eat foods like cottage cheese, yogurt, and blueberries. This is going to last until you are ten pounds away from your goal weight.

During phase three, you will up your carb intake to between 50 and 80 grams of net carbs while you try to find the right balance. This means you have to find how many carbs you can eat before your weight loss stalls? This part has to be done slowly and with some trial and error to find how many carbs you can eat without gaining any weight.

When you have found that number, and have maintained it for one month, you will enter phase four. This will be your lifetime maintenance. This part will focus on keeping up with habits that you created during the third phase. You can consume up to 100 grams of net carbs each day as long as you don't begin gaining weight.

There are many different moving parts when talking about the Atkins diet. With the Keto diet, you can only eat one way for the whole diet. You are going to lower your carb intake to about five percent of your daily calorie intake. Because of this, you will enter Ketosis, and most people monitor this by using a blood test or urine strips.

Many people just recommend the Keto diet for children who have epilepsy because getting rid of a complete food group will drastically change the way you eat, and this might pose some risks. Some evidence suggests that it might help adults who have epilepsy, too. Be careful as there needs to be more research done.

If this diet isn't followed properly and safely, the Keto diet could cause an increased risk of kidney stones and possible heart disease, as well as deficiencies in essential vitamins and minerals. Until your body gets adapted, the buildup of Ketones could cause mental fatigue, bad breath, nausea, and headaches.

You probably will lose some weight with both of these diets. At first, it will just be water weight. There is a chance that water weight might be regained when you begin eating normally again. Studies show that people who followed the Atkins diet lost 4.6 to 10.3 pounds, though they did regain some back by the end of their second year.

Neither the Atkins nor Keto diet makes you count calories. The main thing to make sure of is that you stay under the number of net carbs. Keto does recommend you to be sure you are hitting the right percentage of calories that come from fat and protein.

It all depends on the person as to which diet is the easiest for them to follow. It just depends on your habits before you start this diet. Neither one of them is easy.

The biggest difference between these two diets is the amount of protein you get to eat. Atkins doesn't put a cap on your protein consumption but Keto does. The other difference is having your body in Ketosis during the entire diet. The Keto diet is the only one that requires you to stay in Ketosis. The Atkins diet lets you slowly reintroduce carbs.

This means that the Atkins diet might be a bit more sustainable in the long run since it isn't as restrictive.

A Doctor's Point of View

According to leading cardiologist Dr. Ibal Sebag the Keto diet is a healthy way to lose weight. It is also an effective way to help with some diseases, if it is done the right way and with the help of a qualified health professional. This diet isn't for everybody—and this is why it is recommended to seek the advice of a dietitian or your doctor before beginning the Keto diet. If it was easy to eat nutritious foods and only the number of calories we need to keep us healthy, there wouldn't be diabetes or obesity epidemic. Many people have claimed they have tried every diet out there, and the Keto diet was the only one that worked for them because of the reduced cravings for high carb, processed, and sugary foods. Carry excess weight around the stomach area can increase a person's risk of developing health problems like depression, cancers, sleep apnea, osteoarthritis, stroke, heart disease, and diabetes. For people who have these risks, finding a diet that works is very important.

If you already follow the Keto diet here are some things that Dr. Sebag recommends you do:

1. Talk with a dietitian to make sure your micronutrient requirements are being met. Low carb and high-fat foods often have low water content, antioxidants, fiber, minerals, and vitamins. You have to be careful or you might risk dehydration, electrolyte imbalance, constipation, and vitamin deficiencies. A dietitian will be able to work with you to make sure you are eating the correct foods.

2. Before beginning the Keto diet, talk with your doctor. Get blood work done and know if you are at risk for cardiovascular disease. Your team of doctors can work together to help you achieve your diet and health care goals safely.

3. Try to eat mostly healthy fats such as olive oil, fatty fish, avocados, seeds, and nuts. You need to limit saturated fats.

4. Try to eat vegetables and fruits from every color group each day. Meaning you need to focus on more vegetables than fruits. Look for vegetables that are red, blue/purple, yellow/orange, white/brown, and green. Having a variety of colors will help guard against deficiencies in micronutrients. Make sure you include some foods that contain soluble fiber, legumes, raw nuts, and unsweetened cocoa powder.

5. Stay hydrated. Drink a lot of water. This is an absolute must.

Chapter 1: Ketogenic Lifestyle

Have your friends invited you to go out? Are you afraid to go with them due to food choices?

... Well, you don't have to be. You can eat delicious foods wherever you go.

- Add more good fats.

  Eating at restaurants can be difficult because their meals are usually low in fats. This makes it hard to feel full when you aren't eating carbs. You can handle this in a number of different ways. Ask for some extra butter, and melt it over your vegetables or meat. Ask for vinegar and olive oil-based dressing for salads. Many restaurants serve cheap vegetable oils that are high in omega 6 fatty acids instead of olive oil. People who have been doing the Keto diet will carry a small bottle of olive oil with them.

- Choose drinks wisely.

  The best drinks to choose are unsweetened tea, sparkling water, coffee, and water. If you want to drink alcoholic beverages, stick to dry wine, champagne, or spirits. Ask for them either with club soda (no sugar) or straight.

- Restaurants

  There are many restaurants along with fast food places that offer low-carb options. If you are craving a burger, ask for it to be wrapped in lettuce or leave the bun off. Choosing meats such as steak and fish will keep you in low-carb mode. Never choose any type of potato, rice or beans as a side. And instead, ask for salads, asparagus, and veggies. If you have a Chipotle near you, you can ask for a bowl without rice or beans and have it filled with cheese, meat, sour cream, and guacamole.

- Avoid starchy foods.

Say no to potatoes, pass the bread, bounce on the pasta, and flick the rice. Never allow temptations to get on your plate. Make sure you order your meal without any starchy sides.

When ordering an entrée, many places will let you substitute starchy sides for a salad or extra vegetables. When ordering a sandwich or burger, ask for it to be wrapped in lettuce instead of the bread. If the place won't make any substitutes, don't order the item at all.

If it does get on your plate, figure out your options. If you know you can leave it on your plate without eating it, go for it. If you can't handle the temptation, ask your waiter to replace it with a nonstarchy food. If the place is a casual restaurant, you can just throw it away.

- Be careful with sauces and condiments.

  Sauces contain mostly fats which is okay, however you need to be aware that gravies and ketchup contain mainly carbs. If you don't know what is in a sauce, ask your server what is in it and stay away from them if it has sugar or flour. You could ask them to put the sauce on the side so you can decide how much you want to add.

- Buffets

  This is when things can get tricky. Set some ground rules before you leave the table. Stay away from starches and grains. Go for fats, veggies, and protein.

- Dessert

  If you aren't hungry, ask for a cup of coffee or tea while waiting for your companions to finish. If you are still a bit hungry, see if they have some berries with whipped cream or a cheese plate.

Now that we've covered about what to do when you go out to eat, let's look at the top five restaurants that are Keto-friendly and what you can order.

1. Number Five – Chick-Fil-A

   Chick-fil-A has many low-carb options, especially breakfast. You can get a Keto sandwich and a coffee, and you will be energized until lunch. The grilled chicken nuggets are flavorful but they do have fillers and two carbs per eight nuggets.

   Their avocado lime ranch dressing has three grams of carbs and 32 grams of fat that comes from soybean oil. You might want to stay away from vegetable oil since they can increase inflammation and are full of trans fats.

   Here is a list of their Keto options:

   - Grilled chicken nuggets with a side salad
   - Grilled chicken club sandwich without the bun
   - Grilled chicken sandwich without the bun
   - Bacon, egg, and cheese muffin without the muffin
   - Sausage, egg, and cheese biscuit without the biscuit
   - Bacon, egg, and cheese biscuit without the biscuit

2. Number Four – Kentucky Fried Chicken

   Order your chicken grilled when visiting this restaurant. Their grilled chicken is delicious. You can choose a side with this meal, and their only Keto-friendly option is green beans. The grilled chicken is low in fat so add some fat like olive oil, butter, or avocado to make it filling. Watch out for the "butter" it is actually margarine.

   There are only two Keto options at this restaurant:

   - Green beans
   - Grilled chicken

3. Number Three – Jimmy John's Gourmet Sandwiches

Jimmy John's has a refreshing unwich. They offer a lettuce wrap instead of using bread, and it is really good. It isn't just a few lettuce leaves that are barely holding your fillings together. This is a favorite restaurant with the Keto crowd because their ingredients are fresh and simple.

Here is a list of their Keto-friendly Unwiches:

- Club tuna
- Beach club
- Country club
- Smoked Ham
- Ultimate porker
- Club Lulu
- Bootlegger club
- Hunters club
- Italian nightclub
- Billy club

Ask for a jumbo kosher dill pickle for your side.

4. Number Two – Chipotle

Chipotle is a great Keto restaurant. Their salad bowl comes with lettuce instead of beans and rice, and there is a multitude of options that can be put on top. Try to stay away from their vinaigrette as it is full of sugar. For a creamier kick, add sour cream or queso. If you don't have a Chipotle around and want Mexican, go to Taco Bell and order the Mini Skillet Bowl.

Here is a list of their Keto-friendly toppings:

- Guacamole
- Cheese
- Tomatillo-red chili salsa
- Tomatillo greed chili salsa
- Fresh tomato salsa
- Fajita vegetables

- Sofritas
- Chorizo
- Barbacoa
- Port carnitas
- Steak
- Chicken
- Romaine lettuce

5. Number One – Wendy's

You might not be a fan of fast food burgers, but Wendy's burgers are 100 percent all beef. They don't contain any fillers and are bigger than normal fast food burgers. The ingredients are as good as if you made everything at home.

Here are all the Keto options you can find here:

- Caesar side salad – without croutons
- Southwest avocado chicken salad
- Berry burst chicken salad – instead of ordering raspberry vinaigrette order Caesar or ranch dressing
- Grilled Asiago ranch chicken club sandwich – without the bun
- Grilled chicken sandwich – without honey mustard
- Cheesy cheddar burger – without the bun
- Jr. Bacon cheeseburger – without the bun
- Jr. Hamburger deluxe – without ketchup
- Cheeseburger deluxe – without bun or ketchup
- Bacon deluxe ¾ pound triple – without the bun
- Bacon deluxe ½ pound double – without the bun
- Bacon deluxe ¼ pound single – without the bun
- Son of baconator – without the bun
- Baconator – without the bun
- Dave's triple – without the bun
- Dave's double – without the bun
- Dave's single – without the bun

Five Common Mistakes On The Keto Diet

Looking at It as Just Another Fad Diet

After you have figured out why you want to do the Keto diet, you will need to seriously think about how realistic it will be for your lifestyle. You might need to manage an illness, lose some weight, or fuel for running.

Living the Keto Lifestyle has to be an all or nothing mindset. When you think about the entire system, it is a lot more than just cutting out sugar and bread for a week or so to get your body into Ketosis. It could take from a few weeks to a month for your body to begin using fat for fuel. Your body's natural instinct is to use sugar for its fuel. All your hard work and sacrifice can be undone with just one meal. Keto isn't a diet you can do just during the week and eat whatever you want on the weekends.

If you are using Keto to help you lose weight and restrict your calories, you might regain all of your lost weight if you go off Keto. This holds true if you use Keto to keep you from overeating foods such as cookies and pizza because you are going to overeat these when you decide to stop doing Keto.

If thinking about Keto as a new lifestyle doesn't seem like something you would enjoy, it isn't going to work for you.

Still Consuming Carbs

You may think you have been cutting out carbs, but the truth is they can creep into your diet and knock you out of Ketosis. This happens when you don't measure your portions, aren't keeping track of your carbs, or eat something without looking at the ingredients. Certain supplements and medicines could even up your intake of carbs.

When doing Keto right, it means your intake of carbs per day should be 20 grams or less. To keep you in this range, your carbs need to come from cauliflower, broccoli, and leafy greens. Even these veggies can add up if you aren't careful. One cup of kale has around five grams of net carbs. A kale salad, on the other hand, will weigh in at 20 grams because there are about three or four cups of kale in that salad.

One-fourth of a cup of sweet potatoes has 20 grams of carbs, and one medium apple has 23. Either one of these can max out your carbs for the day.

Incorrectly Managing Your Vegetables

When you think about the issue of carbs, keeping a balanced vegetable intake with this diet is very tricky. When you take the high carb foods such as quinoa, beans, lentils, and sweet potatoes off the table, you are going to have to be creative to build a diet that is balanced with foods that you can eat. If you get rid of all vegetables and concentrate on fat intake, you are leaving yourself open for deficiencies in minerals and vitamins.

To keep your diet nutritious, find your ten most favorite vegetables and look up their net carb content to see if you can put them into your new lifestyle. Try to add leafy greens that are full of nutrients such as spinach and kale into each meal. Always use a food tracker to keep track of your carb intake and watch out for portion sizes. To help with gaps in nutrients, you might want to think about taking a multivitamin.

In the first weeks of doing a Keto diet, and you begin losing weight from water, your electrolyte level might drop, and you may feel a bit crappy. If you experience any muscle problems or fatigue, try taking a supplement such as potassium and magnesium. Avocados, kale, and spinach give you potassium. And oysters, spinach, and hemp seeds will giveyou're your magnesium.

Consuming Large Amounts of Protein

Many fitness enthusiasts and healthy eaters talk about the benefits of a high protein diet, however too much protein is a big no-no with a Keto diet. When you eat too much protein, your body will turn it into glucose, and this can knock you out of Ketosis and back into burning sugar

Keto lets you eat a moderate intake of protein which is about 0.5 to .075 grams of protein for each pound of your body weight each day. If you weigh at 150 pounds this would equal to about 75 to 112 grams of protein every day. Three eggs or a small piece of chicken gives you 20 grams of protein.

Even though you are loading up on fats, you still need to take care of your heart. Protein needs to come from sources such as fish, turkey, and chicken instead of processed foods.

Consuming the Wrong Fats

When you need fat to take up around 80 percent of your total calorie intake, it is way too easy to add butter or coconut oil to everything you put in your mouth. Eating the correct types and maintaining a balance of fats is the key to a healthy Keto diet.

It is critical to get lots of unsaturated fats. Eating fatty foods such as sardines, trout, and salmon; avocados, seeds such as hemp, chia, and flax; and nuts such as pecans, walnuts, and peanuts are all good sources of unsaturated fats. Plant oil such as hemp oil, grapeseed, flax, and avocado are also good sources of unsaturated fats. Unsaturated fats can help reduce the risk of stroke and heart disease.

Self-Discipline and Willpower

There are millions of people out there who want to lose weight. Their biggest challenge is having a lack of self-discipline or willpower. Most people think they can't lose weight because they don't have any self-control. Whatever way you would like to define it, self-control, self-discipline, or willpower is a mysterious and elusive thing. Since the early 1960s, scientists have tried to figure out what self-discipline and willpower is and ways to improve it. People always complain that if they had more self-control they could avoid alcohol, drugs, eat better, exercise more, lose weight, eat more bacon, save for retirement, stop procrastinating, etc. One study showed that around 30 percent of the people they interviewed said their greatest barrier was their lack of willpower when making changes in their lives.

Excellence is a habit.

> Excellence has never been an act. It has always been a habit of repetitive action. In order to understand self-discipline and willpower, you need to understand habit. Habits get created because our brains are always looking for ways to conserve energy. If left alone, our brains would take anything we do and make a habit out of it. It does this to conserve energy and effort. This lets us keep from thinking about normal everyday behaviors such as eating and walking so we can use our mental fuel for more important things such as designing video games, building airplanes, finding bacon, or making weapons.
>
> Our brains will make time-saving patterns during its thought processes in the same way water reacts to dirt. When you drop water onto a mound of dirt, the water will

run off to the side to find the path of least resistance. Every drop will erode a small channel down the side. The more water you drop, the deeper each channel will be carved on this hill. After some time, the water will run down that same channel over and over. In order for the water to go down this channel, the water has to be dropped on the top of the channel. This starting point is its trigger. When the water hits the trigger, it will always go along the same channel. Always.

Habits are our thought channels.

It takes a lot of effort to make water run out of that channel. This is just like our habits. Habits are impulse channels inside our brain that will follow a specific past that leads to the exact same outcome each time without any effort. All this is needed is a trigger. This impulse will follow the channel in our brain without creating a physical or mental routing to happen that will lead to a reward. This is called a habit loop. Basically, your brain has created a trigger that leads to a routine that leads to a reward.

Willpower—what is it?

What exactly is self-discipline and willpower? It's the ability to stay away from unproductive thought patterns. To redirect this habit will take a lot of mental energy. The first studies about willpower give the impression that willpower is a learned skill.

To quote Henry P. Liddon: "What we do upon some great occasion will probably depend on what we already are, and what we are will be the result of previous years of self-discipline." This basically meant that self-control can either be improved or learned. When you repeat a task over and over, it will get easier and take less effort. Therefore, excellence is not an act but a habit of repetition.

This in no way explains why we eat healthy one day and the next; we raid the refrigerator and eat everything in sight. You might be able to exercise on a day without any problems, but the next you can't get out of the bed. Exercising each day wouldn't be hard to do if it was a skill. The problem with the theory of self-discipline is you can't forget a skill.

Willpower is a muscle.

One researcher, Mark Muraven figured out that willpower is more similar to a muscle. He wanted to figure out if willpower were a skill, why can't it stay constant daily?

An experiment was conducted by putting a plate of fresh-baked cookies beside a bowl of radishes. They place the bowls on a table. This closet was set up with a two-way mirror, a toaster oven, a bell, and a chair. They asked for 67 student volunteers and instructed them to skip one meal. Each student filed into the room and sat down at the two bowls. A researcher instructed them that the experiment was about taste perception. This experiment was forcing the student to exert their self-discipline and willpower.

Researchers instructed half of the volunteers to ignore the radishes and eat the cookies. The other half were told to ignore the cookies and eat the radishes. The theory was that it was going to take willpower and mental energy to ignore cookies. It wasn't going to take any energy whatsoever to ignore the radishes when you are staring at a plate full of warm cookies.

The instructor reminded them they could only eat the food they were assigned and left them in the room.

After only five minutes, the volunteers who were allowed to eat cookies were in absolute heaven. The volunteers who were told to eat the radishes were experiencing mental agony.

One researcher reported that one radish eater grabbed a handful of cookies, ate them quickly, and licked any remaining chocolate off their fingers. Another picked up a cookie, smelled it, and placed it back onto the plate. After only five minutes, the radish eater's willpower has been completely exhausted by having to eat a bad tasting vegetable and ignoring a treat. Cookie eaters didn't use any self-discipline at all.

Researchers then went into the room and had the volunteers wait for 15 minutes to allow time for the sensory memory of the food they ate to diminish. In order to pass the time, they were asked to complete a simple puzzle. They were told to trace a shape without lifting their pencil or tracing over a line twice. If they wanted to quit, the researcher left a bell for them to ring. The researcher told them the puzzle shouldn't take them too long to complete. The truth was, the puzzle was impossible to do.

This was the most important part of the experiment. It took great amounts of willpower to continue working on the puzzle, especially after every attempt lead to failure.

What they realized behind their mirror was the cookies eaters had a large reserve of willpower and worked more than 30 minutes on the puzzle even after hitting all the roadblocks.

The radish-eaters with their depleted willpower grumbles showed frustration and complained. Some of them went so far as to shut their eyes and lay their heads down on the desk. One particular person snapped at the researcher when they came back into the room. The radish-eaters only averaged about eight minutes. When they were asked how they felt, one went so far as to say they were completely sick of this dumb experiment.

Cookie Fatigue

When they forced the volunteers to use their self-discipline and willpower to ignore the cookies, it put them in a state of wanting to quit a lot faster. Over 200 studies have been done since this one, and all of them found the same results – willpower is similar to a muscle. It isn't a skill. Willpower can fatigue a person.

This might be why people who choose to have an extramarital affair usually begin them at night after working all day. It is the reason behind why good doctors make stupid mistakes after a long complicated task has taken a lot of intense focus. It is also the reasons why most people will lose control when drinking or cheating on their diet.

Many people feel as if they have no willpower. Self-control and willpower are both learned behaviors that will happen with time. They are also very affected by fatigue. Anybody can have willpower. You have to know how it can be strengthened and weakened.

Intelligence isn't as important as willpower.

One study done in 2005 showed that when it comes to academic success, self-discipline and willpower were more important than how intelligent a person was. It also showed that having better self-discipline lead to less alcoholism, better relationships, higher grades, better self-esteem, and less binge eating. This is great.

Willpower does get stronger the more you use it but has no shelf life. It has to be used daily. It is always stronger during the beginning of the day. It will decline throughout the day as you get more tired.

Ways to Improve This Muscle

The first thing you have to do is write down the motivation or reasons why you want to change. This change must end at a goal. Wanting to lose weight isn't good enough. You need to be motivated due to the consequence of being overweight. Again losing weight isn't a clear goal. You need to set a certain weight you want to get to. You need to write it down legibly along with your reason. For example, "I will lose 50 pounds to help prevent me from getting diabetes." This is a great goal. Self-control and willpower can't happen until these other steps happen. Writing a goal along with two specifics and reading that goal every day will create a trigger by giving the goal specifics.

The next thing you need to do is monitor how you act toward the goal. When trying to lose weight, you need to keep a diet journal. You will need to write down every single thing you drink and eat. Each evening, write out your plan for the next day's meals. That evening, you will audit yourself for either your failures or successes by writing on the same page what you really did drink and eat. Keep doing the same routine every evening. You have to be honest with yourself about why you either failed or succeeded. This last part is what is very powerful. It is called self-introspection. This is the key that lets you see your habits. You will be able to make changes and get rid of any bad habits you see. This helps you strengthen your willpower and form good habits.

Willpower will get strengthened and developed with time. It gets developed by holding yourself accountable for every little thing every day. It has to be written down. If you plan on eating eggs and bacon for breakfast, and you chose something else—why? When you can look at your day, you might realize that you went to bed later than usual and that you didn't get up early enough to cook. So, you choose a yogurt that was readily available in the refrigerator. If you want to have eggs and bacon the next day you have to either fix them the night before, go to bed earlier, or get rid of the yogurt so it won't be a temptation. Planning will reinforce the trigger and gets rid of the mental energy that is needed to have willpower when you don't get enough sleep, feeling too stressed for getting up late, or not having any bacon. It can also give you more willpower to make better decisions during your day. Planning and writing down the next day's tasks gives you strength for willpower in the future and gets rid of fatigue that is needed to make changes the next day.

With time, self-introspection will get easier. It will get to a point that you will do it without even thinking about it. It is the subconscious self-introspection that gets seen by others as willpower and self-control. It is just like exercising to strengthen muscles, writing down small goals and making yourself accountable will make your self-discipline stronger. This self-discipline muscle will get very powerful. With time, you are going to be able to make decisions without really thinking about them. Your stronger willpower will be seen by people around you. You will see that you are just flexing a very well rested self-discipline muscle.

Now you need to attack the hardest decisions during your day in the mornings when you are more energized. These are the things that take the most energy. This gives you more strength to keep your willpower. During the evenings, when your willpower is weak, have some good snack available so you won't be tempted to cheat. Macadamia nuts, guacamole, pork rinds, some pre-cooked bacon, hard cheeses, or rolled meats are all good choices. Learn to make fat bombs and have them handy in the fridge will give you a boost of energy to make better choices when thinking about what you will fix for supper.

Chapter 2: Transitioning to a Keto Diet

You may have seen the word macros when researching the Keto diet but don't have any idea what they are. Well, "Macros" is just short for macronutrients when used in the context of the Keto diet.

Macros are the parts of food that give you fuel and energy. These are protein, carbohydrates, and fats. Your calories come from these. You need to grasp the concept of macros if you want to have a successful Keto diet. They have to be in balance to keep you in Ketosis.

Carbs are the only macro that you don't need to eat to keep you alive. There are essential fatty acids and amino acids. These are the building blocks of fats and proteins. There aren't any essential carbohydrates.

Carbs are made up of two things—sugars and starches. Fiber is looked at as a carb, but while doing a Keto diet, it isn't counted toward your total carb intake. The main reason fiber doesn't get counted is because our bodies don't digest fiber, so it doesn't have any effects on our blood sugar.

This means when you look at a nutrition label, you need to first look for the total carbs and then look for fiber. You need to subtract the amount of fiber from the total number of carbs, and this gives you your net carb count.

Total carbs – fiber = net carbs

This basically means that net carbs only count the sugars and starches in the carbohydrates. When you figure up your macros for a meal, you only use net carbs. You don't use total carbs.

In order for you to succeed, you need to find foods that are naturally low in carbs and the ones that aren't. They aren't going to be obvious. It is obvious that potatoes are high in carbs but did you know that bananas are also high in carbs?

For anyone starting a Keto diet, you need to try and consume about 20 grams of net carbs daily.

Protein is important to our bodies because it will help preserve lean muscle mass, makes hormones and enzymes, the energy source in the absence of carbs, growth, tissue repair, and immune function. Protein plays an important role in our biological processes. Proteins are called the building blocks in a healthy body.

When we eat these, they get broken down into amino acids. Nine of these can't be produced by our bodies. This is why these essential amino acids need to come from our food. These nine includes tryptophan, valine, phenylalanine, threonine, lysine, leucine, histidine, methionine, isoleucine. If there is a deficiency in protein or any of these amino acids, it could cause kwashiorkor, malnutrition, or any other health problems.

When you follow a Keto diet, you need to be sure you eat enough protein to help preserve your lean body mass. The amount you need to eat all depends on your current amount of lean body mass. Here is a guideline:

- 0.7 to 0.8 grams of protein per pound of muscle to help preserve your muscle mass.
- 0.8 to 1.2 grams of protein per pound of muscle to help you increase your muscle mass.

You don't ever want to lose a body mass. You should only gain or preserve. Many people only focus only on losing weight. Many times losing weight mean losing muscle along with fat. Your goal needs to be losing fat and saving your muscles. This is important for people to keep good metabolism.

The main thing is making sure you don't get crazy when you eat protein while following a Keto diet. Too much might put too much stress on your kidneys and could affect Ketosis. Try keeping your macros in the ranges above.

Here is an example:

Let's say you weigh 160 pounds and you have 30 percent body fat. This means you have about 48 pounds of body fat. Then you subtract your body fat from your total weight and this gives you your lean body mass. For this example, it would be 112 pounds.

To figure out how much protein you need to eat, you have to take the lean body mass number and multiply it by the ration from earlier. For this example, you need to eat 89.6 grams of protein every day to preserve your muscle mass. Here is how it looks when written down:

112 pounds of muscle x 0.8 grams of protein = 89.6 grams

The last macro is fat. We need to eat a good amount of fat to help maintain cell membranes, provide protection for organs, absorb specific vitamins, development, energy, and growth. These fats will also help you feel fuller longer.

Dietary fats will get broken down into fatty acids and glycerol. This body can't synthesize two types of fatty acids, so it is very important that you eat them. These fatty acids are linoleic acid and linoleic acid.

These fats are satiating, so it's great for people who want to fight off hunger pangs. Now you need to figure how much fat you need to consume. If your carbs at a minimum, you've already figured out how much protein you should eat, and then the rest of your dietary needs are met with fat.

To maintain your weight, you will eat enough calories from fat to support your regular expenditure. If you want to burn fat, then you will need to eat in a deficit.

You have been given a lot of information to help you figure out your macros, but there is an easier way to figure this out. You can find many different online calculators to help you figure out these numbers without getting a headache. If you would like to use an online calculator, check out the website *Ketogains*. Theirs works great.

Now, if you would like to figure this out on your own, let's continue with the 160 pounds from earlier. Let's say this person is a female, stands 5'4", in her late 20s, and has a desk job. She is mainly sedentary.

Let's plug her into the calculator:

The base metabolic rate would be 1467 kcal.

Daily energy expenditure would be 1614 kcal.

She needs to eat about 90 grams of protein, 20 grams of net carbs, and 86 grams of fat. Her intake is made up of 72 percent fat, 23 percent protein, and 5 percent carbs.

Now you know what macros are and how to figure out your numbers. You are on your way to getting started with a Keto diet.

Foods You Need to Stay Away From

- Sugar – this is the big no-no. You need to stop drinking soft drinks, sports drinks, fruit juices, and vitamin water. Also:

    - Frozen treats
    - Candy
    - Breakfast cereals
    - Sweets
    - Donuts
    - Cakes
    - Chocolate bars
    - Cookies

- Starches:

    - Lentils
    - Porridge
    - Bread
    - Muesli
    - Pasta

- Potato chips
- Rice
- French fries
- Potatoes
- Sweet potatoes
- Beans
- Fruit

- Margarine – you need to use real butter and none of the fake kind.

- Beer – this is nothing but liquid bread.

- Pre-packaged low-carb foods – be sure you read the label before you purchase any of these. Atkins products are not all low-carb.

Trickiest Hidden Carbs

Carbs can be hidden anywhere. Many people think that if you cook your meals and stay away from processed foods, you can say away from all hidden carbs. This isn't true. You might be making tacos at home, including chips and salsa, you are still racking up the exact same carbs as if they were bought from a fast food restaurant.

Hidden carbs like to hide in healthy options such as sugar-free foods.

- Sugar alternatives/alcohols

Sugar alcohols or "the polyols," are in anything that is labeled sugar free or carb free. They aren't zero-carb and some can cause insulin spikes or increased blood sugar levels.

- Molasses
- Yacon syrup
- Agave
- Honey
- Vegetable glycerin

- Spenda
- Maltitol
- Sorbitol
- Xylitol

You can use Erythritol, pure liquid sucralose, or stevia.

- Sauces and Seasonings

You know how to stay away from sweet sauces, but there are other flavorings that can quickly add up to your daily carb count and might be the source of uncalculated carbs. It doesn't matter how delicious and "healthy" these are.

Here is a list of carbs that are in spices, herbs, sauces, and seasonings:

In one tablespoon:

- Paprika – 3.3 grams
- Cayenne – 3 grams
- Oregano – 3.3 grams
- Chili powder – 4.1 grams
- Onion powder – 5.4 grams
- Garlic powder – 6 grams
- Ground cumin – 2.75 grams

Ground/dried less than one grams per teaspoon:

- Coriander
- Black pepper
- Cloves
- Ginger
- Cinnamon
- Basil
- Mint
- Tarragon

Blended spices about one gram per teaspoon:

- Bouillon powders or cubes: one gram per ½ cube
- Pie Spice
- Garam masala
- Chinese 5-spice
- Curry powder
- Any other blended spices just read the label carefully. Look at larger containers if they small ones don't have the information

Fresh

- Lime/lemon juice: 1 gram per tablespoon
- Lime/lemon rind: 1 gram per teaspoon
- Garlic: 1 large clove or 1 teaspoon minced: 1 gram
- Ginger root: 1 gram per tablespoon

Hot sauces, soy sauce, vinegar

- Wine vinegar, cider, and white are all zero-carb.
- Balsamic vinegar: 2 grams per tablespoon
- Balsamic oil, plain: 3 grams per two tablespoons
- Balsamic oil, processed: 9 to 12 grams per two tablespoons
- Red hot or Tabasco sauce has zero carbs
- Soy sauce: .5 grams per teaspoon
- Jamaican, Trinidad, and Cajun read the label carefully.

Extracts or flavor concentrates:

- Orange
- Vanilla
- Almond
- All have .5 grams per teaspoon

Mayonnaise and mustard:

- Dijon or plain: less than .5 grams per teaspoon
- Real mayonnaise: .5 grams per tablespoon

- Protein Bars and Supplements

Anything that is flavored, chewable, or coated are going to be loaded with carbs. If you take two, you have already eaten seven grams of carbs before you ate breakfast. Protein bars are loaded with carbs.

Staying Hydrated

When you are doing a Ketogenic diet, your body will switch its fuel supply from glucose to fat. Insulin levels might become low and fat burning will increase drastically. It will become easy for your body to access your stored fat and then burn it. This is great when trying to lose weight, but there are other benefits, too.

You have to drink a lot of water to make sure you stay hydrated.

Dehydration could cause many problems such as fatigue, cramps, and headaches. Water is extremely important in allowing good health and sustaining life.

Did you realize that it is recommended that you drink in ounces half of your body weight in pounds? Let's say you weigh 160 pounds. This means you need to drink 80 ounces of water each day.

When following a Keto diet, your body will retain less water, gets rid of large amounts of sodium, and your insulin sensitivity will increase. This could cause dehydration.

When your body is getting rid of all the stored glucose it is also losing water. This is why you need to replenish all the water you lose.

- Side Effects of Dehydration

When you are hydrated, it allows your body to get rid of all toxins that enter your body. Dehydration can build up toxins and this can cause many health problems.

Mild dehydration could cause dry skin, dizziness, fatigue, and headaches. When you are taking a long car trip, children don't seem to drink the right amount of water. Yes, this might mean you have to stop more frequently for potty breaks but it is better than your children feeling dizzy and possible fainting.

Severe dehydration could cause major problems such as rapid heartbeat, fever, low blood pressure, and confusion.

- Symptoms of Dehydration

  It isn't always easy to know when you are dehydrated. You need to listen to your body so you can avoid dehydration. Here are some ways you might notice it:

1. The color of your urine: When you look at the color of your urine, you will be able to see if your body needs water. If your urine is darker than the color of a dandelion, it might mean you need to drink more water. Ideally you want your urine to be clear of light, light yellow.

2. Dry mouth or lips: If you notice your mouth is drier than normal, this is telling you your body needs more water.

- How to Prevent Dehydration

  There are several ways you can prevent dehydration:

1. Eat vegetables that are high in water like lettuce, greens, and celery. These could help you become more hydrated. Try to include these in your daily vegetables.

2. Stay away from drinks and foods that promote dehydration: Foods that are high in sodium will cause you to feel dehydrated. Because you are going to be eating more foods with higher sodium content during the Keto diet, it is extremely important to drink lots of water.

3. Coffee: This is a diuretic and could cause dehydration if you drink too much. Adding cream and butter will help increase your fat consumption.

4. Watch out for activities that might cause dehydration: exercising, hiking, walking, running, and other activities that will make you sweat. This removes water from your body and makes hydrating yourself very important.

5. Remain hydrated through the day: You need to create a habit of drinking water more often. It is about you taking care of your health and body. If you have to make a chart that shows eight cups of water and check them off as you drink them. Drink water even if you don't feel thirsty.

Here are some tips to increase hydration through drinking water:

- At home:
    - When you get up every day
    - Before a meal
    - After meals
    - After finishing a chore

- On the go:
    - Each hour when on a long trip
    - Driving home from work or after taking children to school
    - Driving to work or running errands

- At work:
    - Before and after meetings
    - During break times

- When flying:
    - Before meals
    - After meals

- Every hour or so

Here are some ways you can motivate yourself to stay hydrated:

- Add lemon juice to water
- Drink green tea
- Keep water with you at all times
- Drink your water warm if you don't like cold water

When you drink enough water you are going to:

- Help manage your weight
- Keeps your body from getting overheated
- Aids in digestion
- Prevents constipation
- Gets rid of waste through urination and sweat
- Lubricated joints
- Keeps you alert
- Improves concentration
- Keeps your mind sharp
- Reduces headaches

Chapter 3: Apps To Count Your Intake

If you were to ask a group of people who have been following the Keto diet how they keep track of their macros, you are probably going to get different answers. We are going to be looking at two of the most popular apps that are out there. We will talk about how to use each one to track your macros as well as the pros and cons of each. It's important to realize you do not need an app to live Keto, its just helps and makes your life a lot easier.

MyFitnessPal

This is the most popular app out there. It is free if you don't want any of the extra features. This app put an emphasis on social networking and sharing your progress with friends. It also has a huge food database. Basically, any food you eat can be found on this app. Anybody who uses this app can add foods, and this makes it hard to know what food you should choose in their database.

This app doesn't track net carbs. This makes it harder for Keto dieters to use since you have to figure out your own net carbs.

Here are some pros and cons:

Pros:

- Tracking packaged foods that have barcodes
- Large food database
- Social sharing
- Option to add recipes from websites
- Weight gain/loss chart

Cons:

- Doesn't track net carbs
- Inaccurate food database

- Pop up advertisements in the app
- Only uses percentages and not grams

Cronometer

This app costs $2.99. The main differences between the two are the social media and the food database. Its food database is more accurate as it only lists validated entries with details such as amino acids and micronutrients. It app doesn't have to social sharing unless you buy the gold subscription. It does track net carbs where MyFitnessPal doesn't.

Here is a list of pros and cons:

Pros:

- Can interchange micronutrient and macronutrient goals by percentages and grams
- No ads
- Ketogenic diet mod with a net carb tracker
- Better precise food database

Cons:

- Costs $2.99
- No weight gain/loss chart
- Limited food database

Exercising When Doing a Keto Diet

We all know that we have better health when we exercise. If you follow a Keto diet, we know that you will lose some weight. What will happen if you mix the two?

It would be reasonable to assume that when you combine the two it would take your health and weight loss to another level. The truth is a bit more complicated. Since you are already restricting your carbs, there are many changes that might happen and some could even affect your exercise performance.

When you restrict intake of carbs, you are limiting your muscle cells from getting any sugar. This is the fastest fuel source. When your muscles can't access sugar, this impairs their function. High intensity is any activity that lasts longer than ten seconds. The reason for this is that after ten seconds of max effort, the muscles begin to burn glucose for energy through a metabolic pathway known as glycolysis.

Fat and Ketones are not a good substitute for glucose when working out. It is only after you have been working out for two minutes that your body will shift into a metabolic pathway that will use your Ketones and fat.

When you restrict your intake of carbs, you are basically depriving your muscles' cells of sugar that they need to fuel the activities for high-intensity effort for ten seconds to two minutes. This means if you are following a Keto diet, it is going to limit your performance during certain exercises such as:

- Swimming or sprinting for more than ten seconds.
- Weight lifting for more than five reps each set using a weight that is heavy enough to bring you close to failure.
- High-intensity circuit training or interval training.
- Playing a sport that gives you minimal breaks like rugby, lacrosse, and soccer.

This isn't a comprehensive list but it gives you an idea of the kinds of exercises that your body has to use glycolysis for. Remember that the metabolic pathway timing all depends on each individual. There are some people that might maintain performance for 30 seconds without needing carbs.

It is also important that you eat the correct amount of fats and protein when you exercise while following a Keto diet.

Many health professionals, when designing a diet plan, will set the protein intake first Protein always gets top priority because it performs actions that carbs and fats can't. Protein also helps improve satiation, has a better thermic effect, and stimulates muscle synthesis better than other macronutrients. If you don't eat enough protein, you will lose muscle mass and might eat more calories than you should.

If you want to keep your exercise routine or implement one, you need to make sure you eat the correct amounts of macros. Here are a few guidelines:

- Excess calories should come from fats and not protein or carbs.
- Be sure your calorie intake stays in a deficit of about 250 to 500 calories. This is not a priority. Many people don't worry about calories while following a Keto diet.
- Keep your protein intake to around one gram per pound of body weight.

The majority of us aren't athletes and adding in an exercise routine isn't going to be hard. Cardio doesn't require you to exercise at high intensities that require your body to burn sugar and glycogen to get results. You just need to bring up your heart rate and keep it there.

Cardio is a low to moderate intensity and a Keto diet won't impair your performance. You might realize you can work out longer without getting tired when you are in Ketosis.

Here are some examples of good cardio workouts:

- Running
- Aerobic training classes
- Recreational sports
- Swimming
- Circuit training
- Cycling
- Interval training classes

You need to remember that your strength and power might be decreased during these workouts due to carb restriction. If you just want a good cardiovascular workout, it is important that you push yourself to your max strength and power.

Chapter 4: Getting Started

It's important that you understand what foods you can and cannot eat on a Keto diet. Let's go over all of the food that you can eat.

- Meats – You can enjoy all unprocessed meats because they are all low in carbs. If you can afford it, try to buy grass-fed organic meats. Make sure you don't go crazy with meats, though. You are supposed to eat more fats.

- Fish and seafood – All fish, like meats, are a great option. Salmon is the best of both worlds because it's the perfect source of omega 3s.

- Eggs – These are the most versatile foods that you can eat on Keto because you can fix them in many different ways.

- High-fat sauces – These are great ways to get your fat intake, especially if you use coconut oil and butter.

- Above-ground vegetables – You have to make sure that you pick veggies that grow above the ground. The best ones to pick from are:

  - Spinach
  - Zucchini
  - Asparagus
  - Avocado
  - Broccoli
  - Kale
  - Green beans
  - Cauliflower
  - Brussels sprouts

- High-fat dairy – Butter is the best choice here. You should go with real butter and not a tub of margarine. Cheese is another good option. You can eat high-fat yogurts in moderation, however normal milk comes with too much sugar.

- Nuts – These are best eaten in moderation. Carbs can sneak up quickly.

- Berries – These should also be eaten in moderation.

- Water – This is one of the most important things you need to consume.

- Coffee – You either have to consume it black or add some coconut oil and butter.

- Tea – Make sure you don't add sugar.

- Bone broth – This will add electrolytes and nutrients.

Let's Go Shopping

Now that you know what you can eat, you're going to want to shop. Here is a shopping list to help you out, and it's even organized by section.

- Miscellaneous

  - Pork rinds
  - Olives
  - Beef jerky
  - Sugar-free and full-fat dressings
  - Salsa
  - Hot sauce
  - Apple cider vinegar
  - Mustard
  - Pickles – sugar-free
  - Nut Flours
  - Nut butter
  - Nuts
  - Seeds
  - Oils

- Dairy

  - Heavy cream
  - Cheeses
  - Cream cheese
  - Eggs
  - Butter
  - High fat yoghurt

- Fruits

  - Avocados
  - Strawberries
  - Raspberries
  - Blackberries

- Vegetables

  - Zucchini
  - Squashes
  - Garlic
  - Onions
  - Lettuce
  - Broccoli
  - Cauliflower
  - Cabbage
  - Peppers
  - Cucumbers

- Fish

  - Salmon
  - Tuna
  - Shrimp

- Meats

- Ground beef
- Steaks
- Chicken
- Breakfast sausage
- Bacon
- Ground Pork
- Pork Chops
- Ham
- Hot dogs
- Deli Meats
- Pepperoni

Reading Food Labels

You will be finding yourself asking yourself, "Is this Keto?" a lot. We're going to quickly go over how to correctly read a food label so you don't get suckered in by hidden sugars.

First off, let me reiterate that you count net carbs: total carbs-dietary fiber. Alright, let's get started:

1. Read the ingredient list.

    Food manufacturers have to list their ingredients in order of weight. The heaviest is first and lightest is last. If starch or sugar is listed in the first five ingredients, stay away from it. The bad thing is that sugars come in many different names. Make sure you become familiar with sugars aliases.

    Bacon is a tricky one because it's hard to find one with sugar in the first five. There are three no-sugar options. Find brands that write "No Sugar Added" on the pack. Still read the ingredient to make sure they aren't lying. Head to the butcher and ask him to cut pork belly into bacon strips. If you have to pick one with added sugar, make sure the total carbs are zero.

2. What is the serving size?

Serving size is important so that you keep your net carb intake at the right level. Let's take cashews as an example. A serving size of cashews is supposed to be one ounce, which is around 18 pieces according to Google. If you ate those 18 pieces, you would be eating eight grams of carbs.

If you ate the whole bag of cashews, you would be eating 256 grams of carbs. That's way over 20 grams.

Total and net don't quite paint the entire picture because they don't really let you know how many carbs is actually in that container. That's why you have to look at the serving size and how many servings are in the container. This lets you know how much you can eat without going overboard.

Chapter 5: Benefits of the Keto Lifestyle

Anybody getting ready to start a new diet or lifestyle change is going to want to know all of the benefits that come along with it. Throughout this, you will learn about many different positive things that a Keto diet can bring. We are going to look, right now, at what all the hype is around the Ketogenic diet.

- Improves diabetes, obesity, and metabolic syndrome.

  This is the main reason why a lot of people will follow a Ketogenic diet. In all of the reasons we will look at, plus this reason, a Ketogenic diet is perfect for people who suffer from type 1 or type 2 diabetes. It is also perfect for people who are obese because it is able to help them burn off fat, and it spares muscle loss. The Keto diet is able to curb a lot of disorders that tend to happen because of obesity. This includes the symptoms and risk factors known as metabolic syndrome.

- It improves muscle endurance and muscle gain.

  It has been discovered that BHB helps promote muscle gain. When you combine this with a lot of anecdotal evidence through the years, a bodybuilder movement has happened with the Keto diet and how it can help them gain muscle. Ultra-endurance athletes started to use a Keto diet. After an athlete has become fat-adapted, evidence has suggested that their mental and physical performance has improved.

- It can improve eye health.

  The biggest problem that diabetics could end up facing is macular degeneration. It's common knowledge that high blood sugar can end up hurting a person's eyesight and can lead to a higher risk of cataracts. It shouldn't come as a surprise that when you lower your blood sugar levels, you will also improve your vision health and eyes.

- Can stabilize uric acid levels.

  The biggest culprit of gout and kidney stones are high levels of uric acid, calcium, oxalate, and phosphorus. The main cause of this is typically a combination of consuming things that have a lot of alcohol and purines, unlucky genetics, dehydration, obesity, and sugar consumption. The main caveat is that a Ketogenic diet can temporarily raise your uric acid levels, especially if you end up letting yourself become dehydrated. Over time, once you become adapted to the diet, and you make sure you consume enough water, your levels will lower.

- It helps fight against heart disease.

  A Ketogenic diet is able to lower blood pressure and triglyceride level and improve your cholesterol profiles. The reason for this is because of the effects of keeping blood glucose at a low and stable level. While it will likely sound counterintuitive that consuming more fat is going to lower your triglycerides, it has been discovered that too many carbs are the main reason for high triglyceride levels. When you look at HDL and LDL levels, a Keto diet can help raise your good cholesterol and to lower your bad cholesterol.

- Improve your sleep and energy.

  Once people reach day four or five of the diet, many of them report an increase in energy levels and fewer cravings for carbs. The main reason for this is, again, stable insulin levels and an energy source that is readily available for the brain and body tissues. It's still a mystery as to why it helps improve sleep. Studies have found that a

Keto diet helps sleep, as it decreases REM and increases slow-wave sleep patterns. The exact reason behind this is unclear; it probably has to do with the complex biochemical shifts involved in the brain using Ketones for energy combined with body burning fat.

Five Tips for Women

While the Keto diet stays the same for the most part no matter if you're a man or a woman, there are some gender-specific tips that can help you out. That's what the rest of the chapter is going to provide you with.

1. For the first week or so, eat extra fat

   This will do three things. First, it will upregulate your fat burning machinery. It helps your mitochondria to get used to a new fuel source.

   Second, it will make sure that you aren't working from a caloric deficit. It will let your body know you have plenty of food so that you won't go into a starvation mode.

   Third, it gives you a boost, psychologically. It helps you realize that you are able to eat more fat than you thought you could while still losing weight.

   You shouldn't keep eating all of the extra fat until you are trying to put on some weight. As your body gets used to burning Ketones, you can lower your fat intake.

2. Don't work to restrict your calorie intake.

   You know how a benefit of Keto is inadvertently restricting your calories? You shouldn't try to double down on the calorie restriction. Don't believe me. Allow yourself the first three weeks of Keto where you only track your macros. Make sure you are restricting your carbs, but don't keep track of anything else. Don't gorge yourself and don't melt a stick of butter into your coffee. Allow yourself to eat until you are full and then stop. You'll be surprised that you can still lose weight even if you don't track every little thing.

3. Keto and fasting, Remember that you can eat more Carbs.

   Even some men will suffer metabolically when they combine extreme low-carbs with intense fasting. Your calories can get too low for too long. You want to burn fat, but if your body gets too scared that you're not going to get any more food, it might hold onto your fat. By avoiding this , you can up your carbs 5-10%

4. Stay away from nutrient-poor fat bombs.

   Fat bombs are supposed to be your allies to help you through a tough time. Make sure that when you make fat bombs, you do so with the use of nutrient-dense foods. Better yet, grab a salad, olives, nut butter, an egg, and so on.

5. Don't be super strict.

   Making sure you strictly stick to the Keto diet for the first month is great to get you fat-adapted, but after that, you don't have to be so strict. You have created your fat-burning machinery. It's not going to kill you to enjoy a gluten-free cookie your kid surprises you with. Your body is going to bounce back at this point.

Five Tips for Men

1. Try intermittent fasting.

   This is a great way to keep yourself in Ketosis. It would be best to go low-carb and eat at regular times for a couple of days before you start fasting. This will prevent a hypoglycemic episode. This easiest way to fast is to skip breakfast.

2. Eat enough good salts.

For so long we have been told to reduce our sodium intake. But with a Keto diet, your kidneys will release more sodium which can cause a low sodium/potassium ratio. When you are on a Keto diet, you need to make sure that you get an additional three to five grams of sodium. A teaspoon of sea salt will give you around two grams of sodium.

Drinking broth during the day can help you out. Add extra sea salt to your meals is also a good idea. Sea veggies like nori and kelp have high salt content as well.

3. Make sure you exercise regularly.

   Regular exercising will help you activate the glucose transport molecule. This will help you adapt and maintain Ketosis because it will let you handle just a bit more carbs in the diet. Strength training exercises are a good idea and will improve receptor activity. Also, the greater amount of lean muscle you have, the more amount of fat you will burn.

4. Improve the motility of your bowels.

   Constipation is something that most people will face on Keto. Being constipated will knock you out of Ketosis. Eating more fermented foods, drinking a lot of water, adding more sea salt to your diet, and consuming more greens will help.

5. Don't consume too much protein.

   If you eat too much protein, and it would have to be a significant amount, your body can change it into glucose. This will knock you out of Ketosis. Make sure that your fat intake is higher than your protein intake, and everything should be okay.

Meal Plan and Keto on a Budget

A lot of people have the belief that Keto has to be expensive, but that's not true. Since you will be eating more fats, you will feel fuller for longer than you did on carbs, which means you won't eat as many meals. And not eating a bunch of snacks during the day will be its own money-saving tip.

Since you don't have to change your protein intake too much, you shouldn't have to buy a bunch of expensive meats. The following are some good money-saving tips for a Keto diet on a budget:

- Keep everything simple. You don't have to create meals with a bunch of working parts. The fewer ingredients that you cook with, the less money you are going to spend. A simple omelet with a side of water will probably cost you $3.50. A Big Mac would cost $5.

- Use the veggies and fruits that are in season. The rest of the year you can purchase frozen.

- Buying a whole chicken and cutting it apart on your own is usually cheaper. You can also keep the bones to make your own broth.

- Pay close attention to the deals that your supermarket is having and stock up on Keto-friendly items that are on sale, especially if it's something you use a lot of.

It's also a great idea to plan out your meals before you come up with your shopping list. This will keep you organized. Planning out your shopping trips is the best way to make sure you don't spend too much. When shopping, the following things can help you save money:

- Buy regular cheese. You don't need specialty cheeses. Buy in bulk and shred your own cheese at home.

- Skip packaged coleslaw. You can make your own for less.

- Go with simple meats and skip special ones.

- You don't have to get expensive kale. Choose the cheaper greens. They are just as nutritious.

- Cut out excessive nuts because they do add up.

- Pick almond meal instead of almond flour. You can also grind up your own almonds.

- Keep avocados to a minimum when they are out of season.

- Get frozen or canned fish, especially if you like salmon and tuna.

Get the best quality of foods that you are able to afford. Just because everybody believes you have to eat organic doesn't mean you have to. If you're not able to afford it, then do buy it. The main thing to remember is to cook your meals at home and they are going to be healthier, whether they're organic or not.

Also, pick the cheaper cuts of meats, and make sure you check on meats that have been marked down. Cooking all of your meals at home will also be cheaper than purchasing Keto-friendly meals at restaurants. Overall, it's not a big difference picking simple Keto recipes and not the fancy ones that require specialty ingredients.

Quick Meal Plan

Having a good idea of the meals you can eat can help you perform better on a Keto diet. Having options that are budget friendly are even better. Here, you will find nine different meal options separated between morning, lunch, and dinner. Three of these will be really easy on the budget.

Morning:

Bacon and Eggs (Budget Keto):

- 2 eggs

- 2 slices bacon
- Cherry tomatoes

Fry up the bacon and scramble the eggs and serve alongside a few cherry tomatoes.

Pizza Omelet:

- 2 slices bacon
- Basil, salt, pepper
- ½ oz. pepperoni slices
- .5 c shredded mozzarella
- 1 tbsp. heavy cream
- 3 eggs

Fry up the bacon. Beat the eggs, cream, pepper, basil, and salt together and pour into a preheated pan. Allow it to cook until almost done and then lay the pepperoni slices on top. Sprinkle with the cheese and fold the omelet in half. Allow it to cook for a moment and more and serve with the bacon.

Sausage, Egg, and Cheese with Coffee

- 2 oz. breakfast sausage
- 1 tbsp. olive oil
- Slice cheese
- Egg
- Bulletproof coffee

  - 1 tbsp. butter
  - 1 tbsp. coconut oil
  - 1 c hot coffee

Cook the egg sunny side up and cook the sausage in an oiled pan. Lay the sausage on a plate and top with the egg and cheese slice.

Add the ingredients for the coffee to a blender and mix until frothy.

Lunch:

Keto Tuna Plate (Budget Keto):

- Pepper and salt
- Lemon
- .25 c mayonnaise
- .5 avocado
- 5 oz. tuna in oil
- 1 oz. baby spinach
- 2 eggs

Hard boil the eggs and let them cool in some ice water and then peel the eggs. Place the avocado, tuna, spinach, and eggs on a plate. Top with a dollop of mayo and a wedge of lemon.

Cobb Salad:

- 1 tbsp. olive oil
- .5 tsp white vinegar
- .25 avocado
- 2 slices bacon
- 4 oz. chicken
- Hard boil egg
- 1 c spinach

Cook the bacon and then chop up the cooked egg and bacon. Rip up the spinach leaves and top with the other ingredients. Dress with some low-carb bleu cheese or vinaigrette.

Bun-less Butter Burger:

- 1 tsp mayo
- 1 large lettuce leaf
- 1 tbsp. olive oil
- Slice cheese

- 1 tbsp. butter
- Paprika, salt, pepper
- 4 oz. ground beef

Add the seasoning to the ground beef and mix well. Form into two patties. Put the butter in the center of one patty and top with the other. Press together to seal the butter in. Cook until done. Place on a lettuce leaf, do top it with cheese, and do spread on some mayo.

Dinner:

Fried Cabbage with Crispy Bacon (Budget Keto):

- Pepper and salt
- 2 oz. butter
- 1 lb. green cabbage
- 10 oz. bacon

Chop up the bacon and cabbage. Fry the bacon until crispy. Add the butter and cabbage to the pan and cook until golden and soft. Season with some pepper and salt.

Chicken and Mushrooms:

- Handful of spinach
- Pepper, salt
- 1 tsp lemon juice
- .25 c heavy cream
- .25 c water
- 2 tbsp. butter
- 8 oz. mushrooms
- 6 oz. chicken

Add the chicken to a pan and cook until almost done. Allow it to rest as you cook the sauce. Add the butter and mushrooms to the pan, cooking until crisped up. Add in the cream, lemon juice, and water, cooking until thickened. Season with some pepper and salt. Nestle in the chicken and cook until done. Serve with the spinach.

10-Minute Pizza:

- Basil
- 2 tbsp. parmesan
- 1 oz. sliced pepperoni
- .5 c marinara sauce
- 1 c shredded mozzarella

Place half of the mozzarella in a pan. Allow it to cook and melt until browned. Pour in the sauce and spread around. Add on the pepperoni and the remaining cheese. Sprinkle with parmesan and enjoy.

Alcohol on Keto

Alcohol tends to come with a bad rap, and it is one of the most abused substances. It can also cause a big problem for people when dieting, but with self-control and moderation, it can be enjoyed.

If you like to enjoy a few beers, a few glasses of wine, or some shots on the weekends to relax or have a good time, then all is great. But toss in a low-carb diet, and you may find it hard. Most Keto followers will notice that their tolerance drops significantly after they start the diet. And once you find out your favorite drink has 30 grams of carbs, you may think about giving up alcohol altogether. You don't have to throw in the towel right away.

Alcohol can affect a diet in many ways. The first is the way it is metabolized. With a carb-rich diet, your body is busy breaking down sugars, so the alcohol is metabolized slower. On a low-carb diet, your glycogen stores are low and alcohol is metabolized right away. This is what makes you feel drunk.

Another problem with alcohol is that it lowers our inhibitions, which could cause mindless snacking and cheating. You might not realize what you've done until you wake up the next morning with a half of a pizza on your side.

There is also a problem with the fact that you may end up consuming alcohol on an empty stomach, which causes things to happen a lot faster. It's important that you reduce your alcohol consumption because it is just empty calories.

That all being said you are still able to enjoy alcohol in moderation on a Keto diet. Clear liquors at 40% alcohol are safe, and anything that tastes the least bit sweet isn't. Acceptable alcohols are:

- Cognac
- Brandy
- Scotch
- Rum
- Whiskey
- Gin
- Tequila
- Vodka

Wine and beer can still be enjoyed as well. However, you have to know which ones are lower in carbs. Try sticking to dry or semi-dry wines because they have the least amount of sugar. Carb and calorie content also differ based on the brand.

- Red wines:

    - Merlot – 3.7 carbs, 120 calories
    - Pinot noir – 3.4 carbs, 121 calories
    - Cabernet Sauvignon – 3.8 carbs, 120 calories

- White wines:

    - Champagne – 1.5 carbs, 96 calories
    - Riesling – 5.5 carbs, 118 calories
    - Chardonnay – 3.7 carbs, 118 calories
    - Sauvignon blanc – 2.7 carbs, 122 calories
    - Pinot Grigio – 3.2 carbs, 122 calories

There are plenty of low-carb beer options out there, too, if you look for them. Some good examples are:

- Bud light – 6.6 carbs, 110 calories

- Amstel light – 5 carbs, 95 calories
- Coors light – 5 carbs, 102 calories
- Michelob ultra-amber – 3.7 carbs, 114 calories
- Natural light – 3.2 carbs, 95 calories
- Miller Lite – 3.2 carbs, 96 calories
- Bud select – 3.1 carbs, 99 calories
- Michelob ultra – 2.6 carbs, 95 calories
- Rolling rock green light = 2.4 carbs, 92 calories
- MGD – 2.4 carbs, 64 calories
- Bud select 55 – 1.9 carbs, 55 calories

You have to watch out, though. Sugar is hidden everywhere. Gin and tonic have 30 grams of carbs. Tonic water has a high sugar content. If your cocktail comes with simple syrup and artificial lime juice, you are probably at 50 grams of sugar. Stay away from popular drinks and mix-ins.

Sweets on the Keto Diet

A lot of people have a sweet tooth and a Keto diet makes just a bit harder to enjoy sweets. But don't worry that doesn't mean there isn't any hope. There are lots of options of sweets you can make yourself. There are even a few store-bought options, but you have to watch out for hidden sugars with those.

The easiest way to satisfy your sweet cravings is to make your own sweets at home. That way you can control what goes into them. While you can find recipes for cakes and pie crusts out there that are Keto-friendly, they often come with a bunch of confusing instructions and expensive ingredients like psyllium husk powder.

I'm going to share with you some delicious sweets that require just a couple of ingredients and no baking time is required. Something as simple as equal parts nut butter and coconut oil melted together, poured into a greased parchment-lined pan, can make a delicious fudge.

Another fun snack is a three-ingredient coconut bar. Melt a cup of coconut oil and mix in three cups of shredded unsweetened coconut flakes. You can mix in some sugar-free sweetener if you would like. Spread this into a parchment lined baking dish and let it set up.

If you like crunch bars, do melt together 1.5 cups sugar-free chocolate chips, 1 cup peanut butter, 0.5 cup monk fruit syrup, and 0.25 cup coconut oil. Once mixed, stir in 1.5 cups of unsweetened shredded coconut and 1.5 cups of nuts or seeds. Pour this into a parchment lined dish and let set up.

One more quick sweet recipe you can make, melt together 2 cups of sugar-free chocolate hazelnut spread, 0.5 cup monk fruit syrup. Mix in 0.75 cup coconut flour. If it is too crumbly add a bit of water to reach a good consistency. Roll the mixture into bite-sized balls. Refrigerate them for 30 minutes.

Keto sweets are really simple. You can go crazy and make fancy cakes and things. You can simply melt together a few things with coconut oil.

Keto-Friendly Snacks

You will likely not experience hunger during the day that prompts you to turn to snacks, but it still doesn't hurt to have some snacks on hand. Snacks are a good thing to have with you when you are taking a trip to keep from having to find something Keto-friendly at a roadside food joint.

Here are ten great snack foods to keep on hand.

1. Macadamia nuts – these have the highest amount of fat and lowest amount of carbs of the nut family.

2. Pecans – these are a great source of magnesium and protein.

3. Beef jerky – this is a great low-carb, high-fat snack and it's convenient. If you don't make your own, make sure you check the packet to see if there are any added sugars.

4. Half an avocado – sprinkle it with some salt and olive oil and you have a great snack.

5. Smoothie with coconut flakes – a quick blend of protein powder, greens, almond milk, and almond butter topped with some coconut flakes is tasty and good.

6. Cheese and meat roll-ups – in a hurry? Roll up some deli meat and cheese for a quick snack.

7. Charcuterie – meat is a perfect option for a snack on Keto.

8. Olives – grab a jar of olives for a high fat snack.

9. String cheese – all types of cheese is fair game for a quick and easy snack on Keto.

10. Hardboiled eggs – it's easy to cook up a few eggs to have on hand if you need a little something to munch on.

Spices, Dressings, and Sauces

Spices, dressings, and sauces are what can sneak in some carbs to your diet. Spices, specifically, can end up your fat burning process. Let's look at some of the best fat burning, low-carb spices that you should have in your pantry.

- Cayenne pepper – the capsaicin in cayenne can up your metabolism for a short time.

- Cinnamon – cinnamon can fight off carb cravings, promote healthier circulation, reduce LDL levels and blood sugar.

- Mustard seed – spicy mustard works like cayenne pepper and can up your metabolism.

- Turmeric – turmeric and minimize fat and lower cholesterol.

- Garlic – this magic spice can control appetite, fight high cholesterol, lower insulin levels, and lower blood sugar.

- Ginger – much like garlic, ginger can fight cholesterol levels and improve metabolism.

- Black pepper – this spice can up your metabolism and help with nutrient absorption.

- Ginseng – studies have found ginseng can help with weight control.

The only spice you really need to watch out for is garlic powder. The rest you could probably not worry about. There's no sense stressing over 0.1 grams of carbs.

Alright, you're good on spices, so your meals are going to have flavor, but what if they're dry. Nobody wants to have a salad without some dressing. There are a lot of Keto recipes out there where you can make your own ketchup, hummus, and creamy salad dressings, but you can buy some of these things too. The most important thing is to read the nutrition label correctly.

The top five condiments you can buy at the store without too much trouble are:

1. Mayonnaise – check to make sure it is made with a healthy fat.

2. Ranch and Caesar dressings – most of the time they won't be made with healthy fats, but they are great options when you're in a pinch, need to get something quick, or are eating out.

3. Butter or ghee – great for a steak topping.

4. Alfredo sauce – check the label to see if you can find a dairy free option.

5. Hot sauce – most don't have any carbs, but do check just to be on the safe side.

Chapter 6: Maintaining

The only way to make sure you stick with any weight loss plan is to make sure that you are prepared and that you keep track of your success.

Start by removing temptations. Go through your house, and get rid of anything that is not Keto-friendly. Now, this can get tricky if you're not the only one living in your house. This is where you need to sit everybody in the house down and let them know what you are doing. Some of them may want to join you. If there are others that aren't partaking, ask them to hide their snacks that you can't have so that you won't see them all the time. If there are refrigerated things that you can't get rid of because they are somebody else's, get solid boxes to store them in so you don't see them.

When you get snacks and foods, pre-portion them so that you can grab and go and not have to worry about using the right amount. It's easy to sit and mindlessly munch on pork rinds—but that's not good. Put your seeds, nuts, pork rinds, sandwich meat, and so on in serving size bags.

Try to aim for your meals to only contain five net carbs. Also, to make sure you stick to your plan, keep a good journal. Track what you eat and how you exercise—and your moods will help keep you on target.

The important thing is to make a commitment to yourself that you are going to stick with for a certain number of days. At the end of those days, you will reevaluate, create a new goal, and reward yourself. You shouldn't write a timeframe that is an infinite amount of time. It's easier to stick to something if you make your goals small and manageable.

Setting Goals

When you are setting your goals, you want to make sure that they are SMART goals. These are goals that you can feasibly move forward with and start seeing results. The point of your goals is for you to be able to be working towards something that is actually attainable. Using the criteria that I'm going to give you, decide on the things you want to change the most through your Keto diet. Will it fit into the SMART structure? If it does, then you can officially set your goal and start tracking your results.

- S – specific: would anybody that has basic knowledge of the subject be able to understand it?

- M – measurable: are you able to tell how far away you are from reaching it, and will you know when you have obtained it?

- A – achievable: will you be able to eventually reach the goal?

- R – realistic: with your time, resources, and knowledge, will you be able to reach your goal?

- T – trackable: is there an accurate way to track your progress?

Tracking Results

Now you have to figure out how you are going to keep track of your results. You can put in all of your efforts, but if you don't know where you're going and how close you are, it will get confusing and frustrating.

The way you track your goals will depend on what your health goal is. Take a moment to think about the best ways you can measure your progress. How are you going to be able to best see the changes happen not just day-to-day but month-to-month and so on?

The following are some good ways to track progress based on goals.

When your goal is weight loss:

- Take a picture before you start and then take a new picture every month to compare.

- You can do a hydrostatic body-fast test at regular times.

- You can weigh yourself, but make sure that you don't become a slave to the scale. Your body weight will fluctuate daily, and other things like body composition, are better indicators.

- Use a urine test for Ketone levels every day to make sure that you stay in Ketosis.

- Measure yourself. Do measurements of your chest, neck, waist, hips, thighs, and arms before, and then measure yourself again at regular intervals.

When your goal is to improve your mental state:

- Keep a daily journal about how you mentally feel. You can rate your clarity on a scale of one to ten and then explain why you feel that way.

- Track your productivity at work. Write down how much you were able to accomplish, how many projects got finished, or the number of breaks you had to take.

When your goal is better physical performance:

- Keep a daily journal and write down how you feel physically and when you work out. You can also rate your energy level from one to ten before you work out and after.

- Write down the specific results you had at the gym, like distance ran, weight lifted, or the number of reps.

- Keep up with what you ate before and after your workout. Along with your gym results, write down when you ate around your workout schedule.

It's important that you track often. You could feel discouraged from time to time, but if you keep track of your progress, it can keep you motivated. Remember, it's perfectly okay if things don't work out exactly as planned.

Chapter 7: Weight Loss Guide Routine

To help you get started on your journey towards a Keto diet, here is a 30-day meal plan that will help kick-start your diet.

Day 1

Breakfast: Two fried eggs – 1-gram net carb

Lunch: 1/3 cup of hummus with pork rinds – 9 grams of net carb

Dinner: Chicken salad with balsamic vinegar dressing – 6 grams of net carb

Day 2

Breakfast: Two eggs and two slices of bacon – 1-gram net carb

Lunch: An avocado with pork rinds – 2 grams of net carb

Dinner: Tuna salad with two hard boil eggs, bibb lettuce, a half cup of almonds, an apple, and a cucumber – 13 grams of net carb

Day 3

Breakfast: Bulletproof coffee – 0-gram net carb

Lunch: Serving of sunflower seeds – 4 grams of net carbs

Dinner: Two ounces of turkey breast, hard boil egg, a quarter cup of cherry tomatoes, an ounce of sharp cheddar, four pita bites, two tablespoons almonds – 13 grams of net carbs

Day 4

Breakfast: One boiled egg with a tablespoon mayo – 1-gram net carb

Lunch: 1/3 cup of hummus with pork rinds – 9 grams of net carb

Dinner: Chicken salad with balsamic vinegar dressing – 6 grams of net carb

Day 5

Breakfast: Romaine lettuce leaf with a half-ounce of butter, an ounce of cheese, half an avocado, and a cherry tomato – 3 grams of net carb

Lunch: String cheese – 1 gram of net carb

Dinner: Tuna salad with two hard boil eggs, bibb lettuce, a half cup of almonds, an apple, and a cucumber – 13 grams of net carb

Day 6

Breakfast: An avocado with three ounces of deli turkey, an ounce of lettuce, and an ounce and a half of cream cheese – 9 grams of net carb

Lunch: Serving of pork rinds – 0 grams of net carb

Dinner: Chicken salad with balsamic vinegar dressing – 6 grams of net carb

Day 7

Breakfast: Two eggs and two slices of bacon – 1-gram net carb

Lunch: An avocado with pork rinds – 2 grams of net carb

Dinner: Tuna salad with two hard boil eggs, bibb lettuce, a half cup of almonds, an apple, and a cucumber – 13 grams of net carb

Day 8

Breakfast: Two fried eggs – 1-gram net carb

Lunch: 1/3 cup of hummus with pork rinds – 9 grams of net carb

Dinner: Chicken salad with balsamic vinegar dressing – 6 grams of net carb

Day 9

Breakfast: A cup of coffee with four tablespoons heavy cream – 2 grams of net carb

Lunch: An avocado with pork rinds – 2 grams of net carb

Dinner: Two ounces of turkey breast, hard boil egg, a quarter cup of cherry tomatoes, an ounce of sharp cheddar, four pita bites, two tablespoons almonds – 13 grams of net carbs

Day 10

Breakfast: Two hardboiled eggs mashed into three ounces of butter – 1-gram net carb

Lunch: Quest bar – 5 grams of net carb

Dinner: Roll three slices of cheese in three slices of turkey and serve with half of an avocado, cucumber slices, blueberries, and almonds – 13 grams of net carb

Day 11

Breakfast: An avocado with three ounces of deli turkey, an ounce of lettuce, and an ounce and a half of cream cheese – 9 grams of net carb

Lunch: Serving of pork rinds – 0 grams of net carb

Dinner: Chicken salad with balsamic vinegar dressing – 6 grams of net carb

Day 12

Breakfast: An avocado fill with a third of a cup of mayo and three ounces of smoked salmon – 6 grams of net carb

Lunch: Full-fat laughing cow cheese – 1-gram net carb

Dinner: Roll three slices of cheese in three slices of turkey and serve with half of an avocado, cucumber slices, blueberries, and almonds – 13 grams of net carb

Day 13

Breakfast: Two scrambled eggs – 1-gram net carb

Lunch: 1/3 cup of hummus with pork rinds – 9 grams of net carb

Dinner: Chicken salad with balsamic vinegar dressing – 6 grams of net carb

Day 14

Breakfast: Romaine lettuce leaf with a half-ounce of butter, an ounce of cheese, half an avocado, and a cherry tomato – 3 grams of net carb

Lunch: String cheese – 1 gram of net carb

Dinner: Two ounces of turkey breast, hard boil egg, a quarter cup of cherry tomatoes, an ounce of sharp cheddar, four pita bites, two tablespoons almonds – 13 grams of net carbs

Day 15

Breakfast: A cup of coffee with four tablespoons heavy cream – 2 grams of net carb

Lunch: An avocado with pork rinds – 2 grams of net carb

Dinner: Tuna salad with two hard boil eggs, bibb lettuce, a half cup of almonds, an apple, and a cucumber – 13 grams of net carb

Day 16

Breakfast: One boiled eggs with a tablespoon mayo – 1-gram net carb

Lunch: 1/3 cup of hummus with pork rinds – 9 grams of net carb

Dinner: Chicken salad with balsamic vinegar dressing – 6 grams of net carb

Day 17

Breakfast: An avocado with three ounces of deli turkey, an ounce of lettuce, and an ounce and a half of cream cheese – 9 grams of net carb

Lunch: Serving of pork rinds – 0 grams of net carb

Dinner: Roll three slices of cheese in three slices of turkey and serve with half of an avocado, cucumber slices, blueberries, and almonds – 13 grams of net carb

Day 18

Breakfast: Bulletproof coffee – 0-gram net carb

Lunch: Serving of sunflower seeds – 4 grams of net carbs

Dinner: Two ounces of turkey breast, hard boil egg, a quarter cup of cherry tomatoes, an ounce of sharp cheddar, four pita bites, two tablespoons almonds – 13 grams of net carbs

Day 19

Breakfast: Two hardboiled eggs mashed into three ounces of butter – 1-gram net carb

Lunch: An avocado with pork rinds – 2 grams of net carb

Dinner: Tuna salad with two hard boil eggs, bibb lettuce, a half cup of almonds, an apple, and a cucumber – 13 grams of net carb

Day 20

Breakfast: Two fried eggs – 1-gram net carb

Lunch: 1/3 cup of hummus with pork rinds – 9 grams of net carb

Dinner: Chicken salad with balsamic vinegar dressing – 6 grams of net carb

Day 21

Breakfast: Two eggs and two slices of bacon – 1-gram net carb

Lunch: Quest bar – 5 grams of net carb

Dinner: Two ounces of turkey breast, hard boil egg, a quarter cup of cherry tomatoes, an ounce of sharp cheddar, four pita bites, two tablespoons almonds – 13 grams of net carbs

Day 22

Breakfast: A cup of coffee with four tablespoons heavy cream – 2 grams of net carb

Lunch: An avocado with pork rinds – 2 grams of net carb

Dinner: Tuna salad with two hard boil eggs, bibb lettuce, a half cup of almonds, an apple, and a cucumber – 13 grams of net carb

Day 23

Breakfast: An avocado fill with a third of a cup of mayo and three ounces of smoked salmon – 6 grams of net carb

Lunch: Full-fat laughing cow cheese – 1-gram net carb

Dinner: Roll three slices of cheese in three slices of turkey and serve with half of an avocado, cucumber slices, blueberries, and almonds – 13 grams of net carb

Day 24

Breakfast: An avocado with three ounces of deli turkey, an ounce of lettuce, and an ounce and a half of cream cheese – 9 grams of net carb

Lunch: Serving of pork rinds – 0 grams of net carb

Dinner: Chicken salad with balsamic vinegar dressing – 6 grams of net carb

Day 25

Breakfast: Two hardboiled eggs mashed into three ounces of butter – 1-gram net carb

Lunch: Quest bar – 5 grams of net carb

Dinner: Two ounces of turkey breast, hard boil egg, a quarter cup of cherry tomatoes, an ounce of sharp cheddar, four pita bites, two tablespoons almonds – 13 grams of net carbs

Day 26

Breakfast: Two fried eggs – 1-gram net carb

Lunch: 1/3 cup of hummus with pork rinds – 9 grams of net carb

Dinner: Chicken salad with balsamic vinegar dressing – 6 grams of net carb

Day 27

Breakfast: Two scrambled eggs with an avocado and two ounces of smoked salmon – 5 grams of net carb

Lunch: Full-fat laughing cow cheese – 1-gram net carb

Dinner: Tuna salad with two hard boil eggs, bibb lettuce, a half cup of almonds, an apple, and a cucumber – 13 grams of net carb

Day 28

Breakfast: Two scrambled eggs – 1-gram net carb

Lunch: 1/3 cup of hummus with pork rinds – 9 grams of net carb

Dinner: Chicken salad with balsamic vinegar dressing – 6 grams of net carb

Day 29

Breakfast: Romaine lettuce leaf with a half-ounce of butter, an ounce of cheese, half an avocado, and a cherry tomato – 3 grams of net carb

Lunch: String cheese – 1 gram of net carb

Dinner: Two ounces of turkey breast, hard boil egg, a quarter cup of cherry tomatoes, an ounce of sharp cheddar, four pita bites, two tablespoons almonds – 13 grams of net carbs

Day 30

Breakfast: One boiled egg with a tablespoon mayo – 1-gram net carb

Lunch: 1/3 cup of hummus with pork rinds – 9 grams of net carb

Dinner: Chicken salad with balsamic vinegar dressing – 6 grams of net carb

Chapter 8: Ten Most Popular and Tastiest Recipes

Asian Beef Salad

What you will need:

- Ribeye steaks, 2/3 pound
- Chili flakes, 1 teaspoon
- Grated ginger, 1 tablespoon
- Fish sauce, 1 tablespoon
- Olive oil, 1 tablespoon

Salad:

- Sesame seeds, 1 tablespoon
- Cilantro
- Red onion, .5
- Lettuce, 3 ounces
- Cucumber, 2 ounces
- Cherry tomatoes, 3 ounces
- Scallions, 2

Mayo:

- Pepper
- Salt
- Lime juice, .5 tablespoon
- Sesame oil, 1 tablespoon
- Olive oil, .5 c
- Dijon mustard, 1 teaspoon
- Egg yolk

What you will do:

1. Start by mixing the mustard and egg yolk together. As you whisk, slowly add in the olive oil. This can be done either

with an immersion blender or by hand. Once the mayonnaise has become emulsified, add in the sesame oil, spices, and lime juice. Set the mayo to the side.

2. Mix together the olive oil, chili flakes, ginger, and fish sauce—and then add the mixture to a plastic bag. Add the ribeye in and let it marinate together for 15 minutes.

3. Chop up all of the ingredients for the salad, minus the scallions. Split them between two plates.

4. Heat a skillet and add the sesame seeds and allow them to dry roast for a few minutes. Place them to the side.

5. Pat the meat off and fry in the skillet for a few minutes and each side. Cook to your desired doneness, but with this dish, it's best cooked to medium.

6. Fry the scallions for a bit in the skillet.

7. Cut the steak into thin slices. Add the scallions and beef to the top of the vegetables and top with the sesame seeds. Serve with the mayo.

- 7 grams – net carb
- 98 grams – fat
- 34 grams – protein
- 2 servings

Breakfast Sandwich

What you will need:

- Tabasco
- Pepper
- Salt
- Cheddar cheese slices, 2 ounce
- Smoked deli ham, 1 ounce
- Eggs, 4
- Butter, 2 tablespoons

What you will do:

1. Place the butter in a skillet. Fry each of the eggs in the skillet until done to your liking. Make sure you pepper and salt them.

2. The fried eggs are the bread to your sandwich. Add the deli ham and cheese, and then top with a second egg. Sprinkle them with some Tabasco sauce if you want.

- 2 grams – net carb
- 30 grams – fat
- 20 grams – protein
- 2 servings

Meat Pie

What you will need:

- Water, .5 c
- Tomato paste, 4 tablespoons
- Dried oregano, 1 tablespoon
- Pepper
- Salt
- Ground beef, 20 ounces
- Butter, 2 tablespoons
- Chopped garlic clove
- Chopped onion, .5

Crust:

- Water, 4 tablespoons
- Egg
- Olive oil, 3 tablespoons
- Pinch salt
- Baking powder, 1 teaspoon
- Ground psyllium husk powder, 1 tablespoon
- Coconut flour, 4 tablespoons
- Sesame seeds, 4 tablespoons
- Almond flour, .75 c

Topping:

- Shredded cheese, 7 ounces
- Cottage cheese, 8 ounces

What you will do:

1. Start by setting your oven to 350. Add the butter to a skillet and cook the garlic and onion until the onion becomes soft. Add in the beef and cook until browned. Mix in the pepper, oregano, basil, and salt.

89

2. Mix in the tomato paste and water. Turn the heat down and let it simmer for 20 minutes. As this is cooking, take the time to make the crust.

3. Place all of the dough ingredients in a food processor and combine until it forms a ball. This can also be done by hand if you don't have a processor.

4. Grease a springform pan and lay a piece of parchment paper in the bottom. Spread the dough onto the bottom up to the sides with greased fingers. Let this bake for 10 to 15 minutes. Pour the meat mixture into the baked crust.

5. Mix together the topping ingredients and spread them across the meat. Allow the pie to bake for 30 to 40 minutes, or until it becomes golden.

- 7 grams – net carb
- 47 grams – fat
- 38 grams – protein
- 6 servings

Western Omelet

What you will need:

- Diced deli ham, 5 ounces
- Chopped bell pepper, .5
- Chopped onion, .5
- Butter, 2 ounces
- Shredded cheese, 3 ounces
- Pepper
- Salt
- Heavy whipping cream, 2 tablespoons
- Eggs, 6

What you will do:

6. Beat together the eggs, heavy cream, pepper, and salt until frothy. Mix in half of the shredded cheese.

7. Add the butter to a skillet and cook the ham, peppers, and onion. Pour in the egg mixture and cook until almost firm.

8. Turn the heat down and top with the remaining cheese. Fold in half and enjoy.

- 6 grams – net carb
- 58 grams – fat
- 40 grams – protein
- 2 servings

Avocado Hummus

What you will need:

- Pepper, .25 teaspoon
- Salt, .5 teaspoon
- Cumin, .5 teaspoon
- Pressed garlic
- Lemon juice, .5
- Tahini, .25 c
- Sunflower seeds, .25 c
- Olive oil, .5 c
- Cilantro, .5 c
- Avocados, 3

What you will do:

1. Halve the avocados, take out the pits, and spoon out the flesh. Place everything in a blender and mix until completely smooth. Add water, lemon juice, or oil if you need to loosen the mixture bit.

- 4 grams – net carb
- 41 grams – fat
- 5 grams – protein
- 6 servings

Cheeseburger

What you will need:

- Butter, 2 ounces – frying
- Chopped oregano, 2 tablespoons
- Paprika, 2 teaspoons
- Onion powder, 2 teaspoons
- Garlic powder, 2 teaspoons
- Shredded cheese, 7 ounces
- Ground beef, 25 ounces

Salsa:

- Cilantro
- Salt
- Olive oil, 1 tablespoon
- Avocado
- Scallions, 2
- Tomatoes, 2

Toppings:

- Pickled jalapenos, .25 c
- Lettuce, 5 ounces
- Sliced pickles, .5 c
- Dijon mustard, 4 tablespoons
- Cooked bacon, 5 ounces
- Mayonnaise, .75 c

What you will do:

1. Chop all of the ingredients up for the salsa and mix them together. Set to the side.

2. Combine the beef with half the cheese and the all the seasonings. Form into four burgers and cook however you would prefer. Top the burgers with the remaining cheese when they are almost done.

3. Serve the burgers with lettuce, pickle, and mustard. Top with the salsa.

- 8 grams – net carb
- 104 grams – fat
- 54 grams – protein
- 4 servings

Coconut Porridge

What you will need:

- Pinch salt
- Coconut cream, 4 tablespoon
- Pinch ground psyllium husk powder
- Coconut flour, 1 tablespoon
- Egg
- Butter, 1 ounce

What you will do:

4. Place all of your ingredients in a pot. Mix everything together and let it heat over low. Stir this constantly until it reaches your desired texture. Serve this with some coconut milk and berries if you want.

- 4 grams – net carb
- 49 grams – fat
- 9 grams – protein

Bake Brie Cheese

What you will need:

- Pepper
- Salt
- Olive oil, 1 tablespoon
- Rosemary, 1 tablespoon
- Garlic clove
- Pecans, 2 ounces
- Brie Cheese, 9 ounces

What you will do:

1. Set your oven to 400. Lay the cheese on a parchment lined baking sheet.

2. Mince up the herbs and garlic, and chop the nuts. Combine them together with the olive oil. Add in some pepper and salt. Pour this over the cheese and let it bake for ten minutes.

- 1 gram – net carb
- 31 grams – fat
- 14 grams – protein
- 4 servings

Hamburger in Tomato Sauce

What you will need:

Patties:

- Butter, .25 teaspoon
- Olive oil, 1 tablespoon
- Chopped parsley, 2 ounces
- Pepper, .25 teaspoon
- Salt, 1 teaspoon
- Crumbled feta, 3 ounces
- Egg
- Ground beef, 25 ounces

Gravy:

- Pepper
- Salt
- Tomato paste, 2 tablespoons
- Chopped parsley, 1 ounce
- Heavy whipping cream, .75 c

Fried Cabbage:

- Pepper
- Salt
- Butter, 4.25 ounces
- Shredded cabbage, 25 ounces

What you will do:

1. Blend all of the patty ingredients together. Form the mixture into eight patties. Place the oil and butter in a skillet and cook for ten minutes, or until cooked through. Flip them a couple of times while cooking.

2. When almost done, add the whipping cream and tomato paste to the pan. Stir and allow it to simmer for a couple of

minutes. Season with some pepper and salt. Sprinkle everything with parsley before serving.

3. For the cabbage: add the butter to a skillet and fry the cabbage for 15 minutes, or until wilted and browned on the edges. Season with some pepper and salt.

4. Serve the patties with the cabbage.

- 10 grams – net carb
- 78 grams – fat
- 43 grams – protein
- 4 servings

Roast Beef

What you will need:

- Pepper
- Salt
- Olive oil, 2 tablespoons
- Lettuce, 2 ounces
- Dijon mustard, 1 tablespoon
- Mayonnaise, 5 c
- Scallion
- Radishes, 6
- Avocado
- Cheddar cheese, 5 ounces
- Deli roast beef, 7 ounces

What you will do:

5. Lay the radishes, avocado, cheese, and roast beef on two plates. Add on the mustard, onion, and mayonnaise. Serve with some lettuce and drizzle with some olive oil.

- 6 grams – net carb
- 98 grams – fat
- 38 grams – protein
- 2 servings

Chapter 9: Diseases Treated by Keto

The Ketogenic diet has an interesting effect on many different diseases. In this chapter, we are going to quickly look over some of the big diseases that a Keto diet can help combat.

Cancer

The Ketogenic diet is able to starve cancer cells. Otto Warburg, a leading cell biologist, found that cancer cells weren't able to flourish with energy created through cellular respiration but instead needed glucose fermentation. Other cancer researchers, including Dr. Thomas Seyfried, agree and have found that cancer cells can also be fueled from the fermentation of glutamine.

With a Ketogenic diet, you lower carb intake, and it reduces the levels of glucose, which will feed cancer cells. Once your body reaches Ketosis, it will help in depleting the energy supply of cancer cells.

Cancer cells vary from normal cells in many different ways, but one of their traits that is the most interesting regards insulin receptors. On their cellular surface, they have ten times more insulin receptors. This allows cancer cells to fill their self on glucose and nutrients that come from the bloodstream very quickly. As you consume more glucose as your main source of energy, cancer cells are going to continue to spread and thrive. It isn't surprising that the lowest odds of survival in cancer patients are among those that have higher blood sugar levels.

The mitochondria in the cancer cells are damaged—and it lacks the ability to create energy through aerobic respiration. They aren't able to metabolize fatty acids to use for energy. This is the reason why cancer cells thrive in environments that are oxygen-depleted. Instead, cancer cells are able to metabolize amino acids and glucose. Restricting the amino acid glutamine or glucose is important for starving cancer.

Crohn's Disease

Almost every child and adult will experience stomach issues at one time or another, but millions suffer from autoimmune problems like Crohn's disease. These types of digestive diseases, which don't have a medical cure, will require lifetime care for the sufferer.

A Ketogenic diet is able to improve symptoms of Crohn's disease by getting rid of inflammatory foods and gut irritants, like:

- Some high fiber veggies and fruits.
- Dairy
- Refined and processed foods
- Legumes and beans
- Pseudo grains that include buckwheat, quinoa, and amaranth
- Grains like rice, corn, oats, barley, rye, and wheat

With inflammation being reduced, the gastrointestinal system will start to heal. After it has been healed, some people can re-introduce foods that used to trigger their symptoms, like fibrous fruits and veggies, seeds, and nuts.

Diabetes

Duke University Medical Center was one of the first to start investigating how a Ketogenic diet impacts diabetes. They recruited 28 overweight participants who had type 2 diabetes and underwent a 16-week intervention trial.

They had a mean BMI of 42.2 and a mean age of 56. They were all either Caucasian or African American. They consumed a Ketogenic diet where they had to eat less than 20 grams of net carbs each day while they reduced their diabetes medication.

Of the 21 subjects who successfully completed the intervention, the researchers found that they had a 16% decrease in hemoglobin A1c from their baseline. They had an average decrease on 19.2 pounds and their average blood glucose levels went down by 16.6%. In the end, the majority of subjects were able to reduce or discontinue their diabetes medications.

Most studies look at the effects of the Keto diet on type 2 diabetes, but it is still a viable treatment for type 1. There aren't any formal studies examining how the Keto diet affects type 1 diabetics. A study from 2012 did look at the effects of reduced carb diets on type 1 diabetes patients.

In this study, researchers studied 48 subjects with a mean age of 24. For the ones who stuck to the diet, their hemoglobin A1c reduced from 7.7% to 6.4%.

Acne and Skin Problems

Italian researchers, in 2012, published an article that looked at the possible benefits that a Keto diet could have for acne and skin problems. They found that skin problem could be treated in three ways through a Keto diet:

1. It reduces insulin levels. A Keto diet can dramatically reduce insulin levels.

2. By reducing inflammation. Inflammation is the reason why acne becomes so tender, red, and sore.

3. By decreasing IGF-1 levels. The reduction of IGF-1 levels helps regulate sebum production, which can prevent pores from getting clogged.

Depression and Anxiety

You will constantly find stories of how a Ketogenic diet has helped people fight off depression and anxiety. According to Jennifer Wider, MD, says that a Keto diet could cause certain bodily processes that could fight off depression.

Your body produces more GABA, which a major neurotransmitter, while on a Keto diet. When GABA levels are low, you are more likely to experience depression and anxiety. When they are high, it helps stave off these problems.

Weight loss is also able to help relieve symptoms of mental illnesses, especially if one's depression is linked to being overweight.

Alzheimer's Disease

We've always believed that there was no way to reverse Alzheimer's disease, but a Keto diet may be able to help slow down the progress. The brain is an energy hog and demands a constant fuel supply. When a person has dementia, their brain has a hard time burning glucose, which causes sluggish brain activity, brain shrinkage, and death of brain cells.

People with Alzheimer's have an energy crisis on their hands. Luckily, except when Alzheimer's has advanced, the brain does great at burning Ketones.

In one study that placed participants with mild to moderate Alzheimer's on a Keto diet for four months, and had them track the urine Ketones each morning. They had to perform cognitive tests at the beginning, after three months, and then four months later after they had started following their old diet again.

Ten of 15 participants were able to successfully and safely complete the study. The ten that finished had mild Alzheimer's. Those with moderate were not able to finish the study due to caregiver burden.

The cognitive test results in those ten people improved significantly for nine of them. The improvements in their tests disappeared after they returned to their regular diets.

Inflammation and Chronic Pain

Opiates are the most powerful drugs that are used to treat pain, but they pose serious problems and can be addictive. A Ketogenic diet can alleviate pain because of several of its biochemical consequences.

These include the activation of peroxisome proliferator-activated receptors, increased adenosine, decreased neural activity, and decreased reactive oxygen species. Through all of this, a Keto diet can reduce inflammatory and neuropathic pain. Unfortunately, there aren't any actual human or animal tests on the efficacy.

Pregnancy

A big question some women have is if they can follow a Ketogenic diet while pregnant. A lot of people worry that their carb intake will be too low, but there's no real evidence that eating real foods on a Keto diet will harm a fetus.

A lean human body is 74% fat and 26% protein by calories. The human cell's structure is made up of fat and is the preferred fuel source for mitochondria. A fetus will naturally use Ketones before and right after birth.

In the later stages of a pregnancy, there is a greater breakdown of fat deposits, which plays a large part in fetal development. The fetus is able to use transported placental fatty acids, glycerol, and Ketone bodies.

Greater Ketogenesis in a fasted state or with MCT oils will create an easy transference of Ketones to the baby which will let the maternal Ketone bodies reach the baby. Once there, the Ketones are able to be used as fuel for oxidative metabolism.

While pregnant, women will often become more sensitive to carbs because of an evolutionary adaption where they become a bit insulin resistant to allow a good flow of nutrients to travel to the developing fetus.

Breast milk is higher in fat than formula, which is full of sugar and carbs. This means if a baby is breastfed, they will likely be in a Ketosis state most of the time. That makes them Keto-adapted. Ketosis can help a baby's brain develop. This means that it is okay to follow a Ketogenic diet while pregnant.

Chapter 10: Myths and Common Questions

There is a lot of false information surrounding the Ketogenic diet—so much, that many people are afraid to try it. We are going to talk about a few of the most popular myths.

You are only going to lose weight following a Keto diet.

This diet will help people lose weight and burn fat. If you don't want to lose weight, you can still follow the diet to maintain your weight or to help you gain some weight.

Could you really gain weight on this diet? It's possible, if you don't do the diet the right way and never get into Ketosis.

There is a lot of controversy about the low-carb, high-fat diet because some people think you lose weight because of the low-calorie intake. Others think it is because of hormonal changes the diet causes. Many experts agree that it doesn't matter what type of diet somebody does—if your calorie intake exceeds your needs or activity level, you will gain weight instead of losing weight.

If you are eating more calories than you need, even if they come from protein and healthy fats, you will see the number on your scale increase.

If you are not looking to lose weight, should you still do a Keto diet? There are many benefits of the Keto diet that go far beyond weight loss. This diet can help your body normalize blood sugar, regulate hormone production, improve digestive health, improve cognitive function, and possibly reduce the risk of getting heart disease or diabetes.

There's no science to back up the Keto diet.

If you've have paid attention so far, there have been many case studies done looking at the effects of a Ketogenic diet. Specifically, there have been studies done looking at its effects on obesity, cancer, muscle loss, insulin resistance, Alzheimer's disease, type 2 diabetes, dyslipidemia, epilepsy, and high blood pressure.

You lose muscle mass.

The Keto diet can help you gain muscle mass if done correctly. The AHA has claimed that a low-carb diet can cause a person to lose muscle tissue. There are no physiological requirements for your body to have carbs, and as long as you don't let your protein intake slack, you shouldn't lose muscle mass. Your protein intake is what protects your muscles, not carbs.

Exercising is out of the question.

Exercising can help everybody, including ones doing a Keto diet. You might not feel as energized when the body is transitioning into Ketosis but this will lessen as your body adjusts. Even during high-intensity workouts, won't cause your performance to decline.

You do not need to stop working out while on the Keto diet. You might have to modify your workouts a bit. If you can handle it, exercising while in Ketosis will burn fat two to three times faster. It can also maintain blood glucose levels and you will notice less fatigue with activity.

To make sure you help your body during workouts, you need to eat enough calories including those from fat. Make sure you let your body recover between tough workouts.

If you find yourself struggling very bad while working out and having a hard time recovering, then try eating more carbs just before exercising. If you fast while on the Keto diet, save your high-intensity workout for times when you are more fueled up.

Everybody will suffer from the Keto flu.

Everybody is going to react differently when their body adapts to Ketosis. This makes it hard to figure what a person is going to experience, how severe their reactions are going to be, and how long it will last. Some transition more smoothly than others. Some may experience fatigue, brain fog, sleep problems, and digestive problems for the week after they reach Ketosis. Keep in mind, these are only temporary problems and will go away with time, with more water, or with more salt.

You can eat all types of fat as people do on Atkin's.

Even though the majority of your calories should come from fat, this doesn't mean you should consume all the saturated fats that you want. Keto diet wants you to eat healthy fats, whereas the Atkin's diet allows all types of fatty foods. A lot of people who follow a Keto diet will stay away from processed meats like bacon, sausage, and salami.

You also have the option of eating clean on Keto and avoiding cheeses, bad quality meats, trans fats, fast food, fried foods, and processed foods. Most people who follow a Keto diet will turn towards healthier options like EVOO, coconut oil, grass-fed butter and meats, nuts, avocados, wild caught fish, pasture-raised poultry, and organic eggs.

Keto is dangerous.

As with anything in life, there are downsides to a Keto diet, but it's not dangerous. Most bad things like kidney stones, increased risk of heart disease, vitamin and mineral deficiencies, high cholesterol, decreased bone density, and gastrointestinal distress can be reduced with water and supplements.

As long you as you make sure you are getting plenty of electrolytes and water, you shouldn't have a problem.

10 Important Questions

Now that we have gotten the myths out of the way, let's look at the ten most popular questions concerning the Ketogenic diet.

1. How soon will I hit Ketosis?

   You have to allow your body enough time to adjust to the diet. This means you have to be strict with your carb intake. If you can't remain consistent, then you may not ever reach Ketosis. That said, if you stay consistent, reaching Ketosis can take anywhere from two to seven days. It will all depend on the foods you eat, your body type, and activity level.

2. Do I need to count calories?

   Yes, calories do matter. Calories are what will affect if you lose weight or not, so you do need to eat in a deficit of calories in versus calories out. But, with a Keto diet, calories don't tend to be as much of a concern. Fats and protein will make up most of your diet, and it will take fewer calories to make you feel full than with a diet high in carbs.

3. Can I eat too much fat?

   Yes, you could end up eating too much fat. This goes back to the calories. You have to make sure you keep your calories in a deficit, so it is possible to consume too many calories from fat. This is why you should keep a macro and calorie tracker on your phone so that you can put in the foods that you eat. You will be less likely to over-consume that way.

4. Should I take supplements?

   It's not a bad idea to start taking supplements since you will be cutting out food sources that would naturally provide with these vitamins and minerals. Start taking them especially if you start to feel crampy or just unusual once you start your diet. The following supplements can help you:

   - Potassium
   - Vitamin D
   - Vitamin B complex
   - Magnesium
   - Multivitamin for men
   - Multivitamin for women

   Make sure that you talk to your doctor first if you are on any other medications because there could be an interaction.

5. Should I worry if I exercise?

   No. Exercising is completely safe on a Keto diet, as we discussed earlier. But a Keto diet can affect the way you exercise. If you do a lot of cardio work like running, biking, dancing, and so on, then you can get away with a little more carbs. If you like to lift weights, then you may have to adjust your goals. Carbs do help with muscle performance and recovery. That's why a lot of strength trainers will follow a cyclical or targeted Ketogenic diet, meaning the up their carb intake right before a weight session. You don't have to do this, though. You may just have to lower your weight the number of reps and sets you perform.

6. I've stalled in my weight loss, what now?

   Everybody will probably hit a plateau on any diet. There are a lot of things that could cause this, but there are just as many things to help you work through it. Here are a few suggestions:

- Switch to measuring yourself instead of weighing
- Cut out processed food.
- Check food labels for hidden carbs.
- Cut out some artificial sweeteners.
- Cut out nuts.
- Lower your carb intake.
- Increase your fat intake.
- Quit eating dairy.

7. I'm constipated, what should I do?

It's not uncommon for people who start a Keto diet to have irregular bowel movements. The following list is a few things that you can do to fix you bowel problems:

- Add a magnesium supplement
- Up your water consumption
- Drink coffee or tea
- Eat chia or flax seeds
- Consume more veggies that have high fiber content
- If you eat a lot of nuts, quit
- Try consuming a tablespoon of coconut oil

8. What do I do if I feel crampy?

Headaches and brain fog is a common issue for people who are just starting a Keto diet. Since you will urinate a lot more, you will lose a lot of water. Add that to all the fat burning that will be happening, and you have a recipe for disaster. Urinating more will cause a loss of electrolytes and you have to replace these. Add more salt and water to your diet to combat this problem.

9. How can I tell if I'm in Ketosis?

A lot of people will use *Ketostix* to figure out if they are in Ketosis. These are available online and in most pharmacies, but they aren't completely accurate. You will urinate on them each morning and if they turn purple or pink, you are producing enough Ketones. If it comes out darker than that, then you are probably dehydrated and you Ketone levels are really concentrated.

10. Am I going to lose a lot of weight?

How much weight you lose will depend on you. Exercising can help you lose more. If you completely cut out wheat products, dairy, and artificial sweeteners, you will probably lose more. Just know that first big drop in weight that you will experience after a week or two is mainly water weight. You probably haven't burned that much fat yet. Ketosis has a diuretic effect on the body. The next drop will be fat as long as you have remained in Ketosis.

Chapter 11: Popular Keto Celebrities and Athletes

Vanessa Hudgens

Vanessa Hudgens has taken charge of her career and her diet—and through the Keto diet, she's gotten the best shape of her life. The star has removed refined sugars, dairy, and carbs from her diet. Since she started the Ketogenic diet, Vanessa has dropped ten pounds.

The key to her success was avocados. She made sure to eat one per day. She explained, "If I'm not getting enough, my body holds on to calories. We've been trained to think that fats are bad, but they're so good."

She adds Soul Cycling to her routine as well. When she worked to drop the 20 pounds she had to put on for her movie *Gimme Shelter*, she liked grabbing a front-row seat. This gave her the motivation to pedal faster. She makes sure to grab a class when she can, and she also does circuit training and Pilates.

Vanessa starts her down out with half an avocado, bacon, and eggs—and as the day progresses, she balances her healthy fats and protein with lots of produce. She normally has a salad with dark meat chicken for lunch with a half of an avocado. For dinner, she usually has a grilled steak or salmon with sautéed veggies.

She also tops her diet with some detox teas. She specifically uses Flat Tummy Tea for 28 days to help combat bloating. She rounds out her healthy Ketogenic diet with yoga. Yoga is what helps her center herself after she films an intense movie.

LeBron James and Ray Allen

LeBron adopted a Ketogenic-style Paleo diet a few years back, eliminated nearly all carbs, sugar, and dairy. He followed the strict diet for 67 and said he did so to test his "mental fortitude" and his willpower. During this time, his diet consisted of low-sugar fruits, vegetables, fish, and meat.

For lunch, he liked to have salads. He shared a couple of his meals on Instagram. One was an arugula salad topped with cashews, mangoes, strawberries, and chicken, with a light vinaigrette. Another one of his meals with lobster salad and mango chutney.

LeBron has never come out and said how much weight he lost exactly, but Brain Windhorst, an ESPN reporter who has a lot of access to James, estimated his weight loss to be anywhere from 12 to 20 pounds.

The 6'8" basketball star weighed around 270 the season prior to his Keto diet. The following season, he was down to 250. LeBron had been inspired by the transformation of his former Miami Heat teammate, Ray Allen. Ray had gotten super-fit when he switched to a low-carb Paleo diet during the summer of 2013.

Allen had come back after the summer break a lot better shape than he had been the year before after he adopted his sugar-free, low-carb Paleo diet. Allen didn't start the diet for weight loss. He said that his new diet provided him with more stamina and improves is workout recovery. He also motivated Dwayne Wade.

Ohio State University professor and dietitian, Dr. Jeff Volek, said James' weight loss was because of his Ketogenic-inspired eating plan. Volek explained that many athletes have started to favor high-fat, low-carb diets to lose weight fast and change how their fat composition.

Halle Berry

At 51, Halle Berry looks amazing and does that with the help of a Ketogenic diet and great genetics. She follows a Keto diet for weight management and to manage her diabetes, which she was diagnosed with at 22.

Following the very low-carb, moderate-protein, and high-fat encourages her to burn fats instead of carbs for energy. Halle fills up on butter, coconut oil, and avocado.

In an interview with PeopleTV, she explained that legumes, nuts, protein, and eggs also made their way onto her plate along with lots of veggies. She explained that it was far from deprivation. She said, "You can eat all the food you want. You can eat a big-ass porterhouse steak if you want. You just can't have the baked potato."

You can easily see all of her favorite meals on her Instagram page. She also finds inspiration from Maria Emmerich. Here's what Halle's typical day looks like:

- Breakfast – Bulletproof collagen protein or greens and beets.

- Lunch – prosciutto and arugula roll-ups or green beans and Bolognese

- Dinner – instant pot white chicken chili or arctic char with olive salsa

- Snacks – tomato tulips, chicken bone broth, or zucchini chips

The Ketogenic diet is definitely working for Halle, and it is a perfect way to help her with her diabetes.

Conclusion

Congratulations of finishing the Modern Ketogenic Diet.

Taking the first steps toward a healthy life is one of the hardest and bravest things that people can do. By choosing to try a Keto diet, you are making that step. Use the information you have learned to make the transition easier and more fulfilling. The best place to start would probably be by figuring out your macros and then going through your house and cleaning out Keto-unfriendly foods.

This won't be the easiest thing you have done in life, but it will be fulfilling. You will notice changes quickly, and if you stick to your macros, you will see the weight fall off. You can enjoy the diet. With a little creativity, you can enjoy the most delicious meals you've ever had, and you won't feel like you're missing out on anything.

Make sure that you have your goals set and have all of the foods you need to be a success. Make sure that you have plenty of fats because that will be what keeps you full. Snacks may also be a great option. Play around with your macros to figure out what works for you. The important thing is that you make this diet work for you. Now, go get started.

Finally, if you found this book useful in any way, a review on Amazon is always appreciated!

www.ingramcontent.com/pod-product-compliance
Lightning Source LLC
Chambersburg PA
CBHW072149020426
42334CB00018B/1933